MW00835266

HOPE
ETERNAL

Rebecca Lynn

ISBN 978-1-64468-559-4 (Paperback)
ISBN 978-1-64468-560-0 (Digital)

Copyright © 2020 Rebecca Lynn
All rights reserved
First Edition

All rights reserved. No part of this publication may be reproduced, distributed, or transmitted in any form or by any means, including photocopying, recording, or other electronic or mechanical methods without the prior written permission of the publisher. For permission requests, solicit the publisher via the address below.

Covenant Books, Inc.
11661 Hwy 707
Murrells Inlet, SC 29576
www.covenantbooks.com

DEDICATION

This book is dedicated to my children.
We all went through this journey together.
Thank you for all of your love and support.

Love,
Mom

CHAPTER 1

"Mom, am I past the part where I could die?"

Kyle Robert's question weighed heavily in my heart as I sat alone in his dark hospital room. He looked very peaceful as he lay there sleeping. I glanced up at the clock, which was registering 2:00 a.m. It was July 22, 2007, and it had been about twelve hours since we entered the emergency room at University of Michigan Hospital, in Ann Arbor, Michigan.

My mind wandered back to Kyle's question, not that he asked it during this hospital trip, but back in May 2006, following his surgery and the completion of three rounds of very harsh chemotherapy sessions. Kyle had approached me in the kitchen and had a very serious look on his face as he asked me this question. He didn't want to continue with the cancer treatments; after all, they said they had removed 99 percent of the cancer from his body. Oh, as a mom, I wanted to tell him 100 percent that he was past the part where he could die. But because I am a realist mom, I had to share with him that I didn't know if he was past the part where he could die. I decided to shake my thoughts and remember where we were just a couple of days ago. He had been enjoying the carefree life of a teenager for the first time in eighteen months!

He had been lazily swimming and doing cannonballs to entertain his little brother in the hot Texas sun. They were laughing and giggling and trying to out-splash each other. As I watched them playfully romp in the pool, I thought about how this summer and the next few months might play out and how through Kyle's eyes they must look so inviting!

Most would agree that a typical fifteen-year-old teenager enjoys a summer that might include such things as sleeping in, running with friends, camping, swimming, and perhaps taking driver's education or visiting family in another state. Teenagers are generally carefree and rarely think about serious things or situations. I was thinking of some questions I thought of asking him. Did he see a brand-new beginning? A new beginning where one time he questioned if he would ever have a future again? Was swimming, which was once taken for granted, now a precious gift? How about just walking in public without worrying about the germs that one may catch that could potentially be life threatening? Perhaps he saw a schedule that was void of appointments, especially doctor and hospital appointments. What about looking forward to the coming school year with such anticipation that one would think it was his first day of school ever?

As I refocused on my son jumping for the umpteenth time into the pool, making cannonball splashes to entertain his little brother, I thought long about these carefree days of summer. I not only wondered what may be going through his mind, but I tried to look through the eyes of my son. I tried to envision how life was anew for him, exciting, challenging and full of anticipation on what the future might hold. He couldn't' wait for school to begin, but not until he was able to enjoy so many "normal" pleasures he had missed out on over the last year and a half. Of that I was certain.

You see, he was a cancer survivor! He had faced the battle that we lovingly called our cancer journey and was now experiencing being cancer-free! He hadn't been able to swim because of his central line, which was place on his chest on a day in February 2006 just two weeks after discovery of the tumors that engulfed his abdomen. He wasn't able to participate in sports and rarely walked the mall, shopped, or even went to see a movie unless it was during the slower, less-crowded times. When he was allowed to go out, he was generally seen in public wearing his green industrial mask, which covered his mouth and nose. We had to be so careful that he didn't pick up any germs that just might land him in the hospital with a life-threatening illness—well, at least life-threatening to an immune-compromised individual.

This hot day in Texas, there was no mask or central line to inhibit the fun the boys were having. It was so nice to listen to the giggles and laughter and watch their splashes and horseplay. My heart just sang with joy! I praised the Lord that we had made it through these last eighteen months with His love, help, and strength. I watched Kyle mature as a man and as a Christian. The trust he showed in the Lord, the medical staff, and me was totally amazing. Kyle didn't realize it, but he taught me about trust and acceptance. We had a plan, and that was that I took care of all the medical and he did as he was asked. He trusted without question. I saw a childlike faith in my son, a faith that I came to understand throughout our cancer journey. I was so touched by his trust that I longed to be able to trust someone in that capacity. We trusted the information the medical staff shared about Kyle's cancer and the treatment they were going to be using. I had trusted people—my pastor, family, and some of the fellow parents and staff on C.S. Mott Children's Hospital, 7th Floor, referred to as either Mott 7, or 7 Mott that I grew to know. I had tried to trust the way Kyle did but learned very soon that even though humans are around, they may not be readily available when I needed them for support. So I turned to the Lord, reading His work, working in Bible study workbooks, studying devotionals, and praying. I knew the Lord personally, but this journey really taught me what it meant to be truly one with Him.

For me, prayer can be just one word, *help*, or perhaps a phrase like "Thank you for walking with me today, Jesus" or even just the act of writing praises, fears, joys, and worries in a journal. No matter when or how I talked to the Lord, I somehow instilled that in Kyle, I guess, by example. I realized rather quickly that I would be alone in this journey in so many aspects. People would care, while others would dismiss us, not wanting to hear about our trials; but God never left us. In fact, He just grew stronger in both of our hearts and daily living.

There was one day in particular when Kyle wasn't feeling well during a very rough moment. I suggested he pray. We were a family that had prayed together on several occasions. Dinner-time prayer, bedtime prayers, or even thanksgiving prayers were not foreign to us. However, we did not truly understand what it meant to "pray without ceasing." We soon learned what that scripture verse meant. We would pray throughout the day and night at all times—in all circumstances. Prayer calmed Kyle down, and from that day forward, all he would do is pray to receive comfort, and I could see the peace of the Lord wrap him up like a child in their mother's arms.

As the mother of these two boys and four other children, I knew what it meant to wrap my arms around them with love. I adoringly watched as my two sons climbed out of the pool and decided it was time to get out of the hot Texas sun. Even the pool water was "almost too warm," they had exclaimed.

Kyle grabbed his towel, took his five-year-old brother Christian's hand and began the trek back to the condominium where their sister, Gina Brienne, lived. He was talking about how they would swim again later and the restaurants we would visit while there. He expressed that he was tired and thought a nap was in order for both of them.

Kyle looked drained. His coloring hadn't come back to precancerous days yet because the effects of all the treatments were still wreaking havoc with his body. The doctor had just given us a 'script for Celebrex but suggested we wait for him to begin taking it until after our trip. It can cause bowel-irritation difficulties, and he did not need to worry about that while enjoying his vacation. His blood counts were still lower than the "normal" person's counts. I thought, "Man, that radiation had zapped him good back in the fall." He was still trying to eat and gain weight, but his appetite hadn't increased as of yet.

Naps became a normal afternoon routine. Kyle tried to eat lunch, but he became full very quickly. He promised to eat more when he woke up. I always admired him. He was so accepting of the whole cancer situation, and he did as he was asked. He ate, actually he drank, "food" that would be difficult for anyone to swallow, and he usually did it with a smile or with some kind of a joke to share.

You see, I was a little overprotective these past few days. Funny, my family and Kyle would tell you that I was always overprotective, and maybe so. Anyway, I was more so since his seizure occurred on our trip down to Texas from Michigan. On July 2, 2007, I was awakened to the sound of rubbing on the bed sheets. I noticed Kyle's head was hanging over the bed and his body was shaking violently. It is not something I can easily erase from my memory.

"Oh, Mom, I'm fine," he told me after he became alert, which really happened once the ambulance arrived at the hospital. He was wiggling his feet back and forth as we talked. His emergency-room nurse entered the room, quickly pulling the curtain back to see Kyle. She had a look of panic and then relief when she saw us talking and smiling. She then explained how she could only see his feet moving and thought he was having another seizure. She politely asked him not to do that anymore. He asked, "What, this?" and he jiggled his feet while laughing. Then he promised he wouldn't do it again and that he was sorry he scared her for absolutely no reason. I just shook my head and relief came over me. My boy was back on track once again!

They had ordered a CT scan to see if they could determine a cause for the seizure, but the scan was clean, which means no evidence of anything abnormal. Perhaps, I thought, it was the chemo he had taken that was just messing with his nervous system. After all they, had used some pretty potent medication during his treatments. Each patient may react a little differently to the chemotherapy received. Plus, we had to add outrageous amounts of radiation that were administered to his entire chest, abdomen, and pelvis as part of his protocol. No one knew what all the side effects would possibly be!

We were eventually released from the hospital and continued on our journey south. We would seek the doctor's opinions and advice when we returned from vacation, but for now we were going to enjoy our vacation and maintain a close watch on any headaches he continued to mention. We all decided at this point that it was probably side effects from the medications.

Accepting the idea that the medication may have messed with him, he joked about it every opportunity he could. Things were happenings within his body that just didn't make sense. He was walking when suddenly he fell near the sidewalk. "Oh, Mom, I just tripped," was his response. I wanted him to stay home, but he was not having any part of that idea! He was off to the store with Gina and probably to a movie too. He was excited for the fireworks later that evening. Anything to do with fire, in any capacity, intrigued him. He had talked about how he couldn't wait to go camping next month when his third oldest sister, Anneliese, was getting married. Cabins, Lake Huron, and campfires! He designated himself the keeper of the fire for the event. So staying home because he had tripped and was slightly tired was totally out of the question. He accepted he didn't feel up to par, but there was no stopping him! He was a teenager on the loose, with places to see, things to do, and life to live!

Kyle amazed so many that knew him. He had accepted his diagnosis of cancer with a very calm attitude. He was only thirteen when they found the tumors that encompassed his lower abdomen and one-third of this liver. Each time they thought they had a diagnosis, actually three times before the lab work finally matched 100 percent, he said, "Okay, what do we do next?" When the final and correct diagnosis was presented, he said, "Well, at least I can pronounce this one!"

Desmoplastic small round cell tumor—yes, this was the name of his type of cancer, DSRCT for short. It is also known as desmoplastic small blue round cell tumor. Upon receiving this news, the protocol began for treatment, and it was to take nearly a year to complete if he stayed on schedule.

December 2006, he had asked me to stop telling people that he had cancer because "Mom. It's gone." He was correct! The January 2007 scan revealed *no* cancer—news every patient and parent long to hear! And absolutely correct he had been! Trust me, I heard about it in the most playful way when the scan came back, all clear! He smiled at me with a very infectious smile during that office visit. I could just hear it in his voice, that "I told you so!" The joy was shining in his beautiful blue eyes. Oh, what a happy day!

Kyle amazed me. He just accepted every step of this journey. Very few questions and very few complaints ever escaped his lips. He was being very accepting again while we were in Texas. After falling a few more times and experiencing continuous headaches, I suggested we go to the local hospital in Round Rock, Texas. I thought he needed to just get checked out again. He was in agreement and quietly lay on the examination table waiting for the doctor to come in. He had expressed to me that he never used to get headaches and asked, "Is this what your migraines feel like?" I shared that no headache was fun and hopefully we could figure out what was going on with him so they would go away. They determined he was still having seizures, but they were not breaking through completely. The plan was to increase his antiseizure medication and hope that this would help the headaches disappear until he could go to U of M for further examination and follow up.

As a mom, I didn't have a good feeling about this newest development. Kyle was so positive; and even though his head was hurting, his back was sore, and he was not able to move his legs the way he'd like sometimes, he just continued to accept each step of the journey. Once the medication was increased, he didn't mention the headaches very often, but his boney back made it difficult to get comfortable. He tried to eat but just didn't have much of an appetite.

After nearly two weeks since arriving in Texas, Kyle fell down the stairs, "Mom, I think it's time for us to go home." It was July 18, 2007, and he accepted the fact that something was wrong. He was ready to end our stay early so we could get back to the doctors at University of Michigan C. S. Mott Children's Hospital in Ann Arbor.

Three days later, as I was pushing my son on the wheelchair into the emergency room at U of M, my mind went back to two of my son's comments over the course of our journey, "Mom, am I past the time where I could die?" and "Mom, remember God has a plan, and He is in control." Kyle looked up at me and smiled, as though he could read my mind. The sliding doors opened; the next phase of our lives was about to begin. We entered the hospital with an understanding that we would accept the next path God had planned for Kyle's life, actually our lives. I was soon brought back to reality as the bedroom door opened, letting a stream of light enter from the dimly lit hallway.

The moment of truth was at hand as two white coats, as I lovingly referred to the student doctors, quietly walked into the darkened room. I sat up and looked into their eyes and watched their faces. They glanced at Kyle, who was still asleep, and approached me.

"We have the results from Kyle's MRI."

I knew our path was laid before us, and either way, the path would lead to *life*.

"The results reveal…"

CHAPTER 2

Did you think it was going to be that easy? I mean, that you would learn the results without a trip down memory lane first? You see, I must go back to January 26, 2006. This is the day our world changed forever!

It all began with the ringing of the alarm at 6:30 a.m. It was time for Kyle to awaken for school. He hadn't meandered upstairs yet, so I went to the top of the stairs and called down to him, "Rise and shine!"

He replied, "Okay, Mom, I'm up."

He hadn't been feeling well the past couple of days, so I was anxious to see how his night went. He had stayed home from school the day before, which was very unusual since he had held perfect attendance for over three years. His right side had been hurting off and on, but yesterday it was compounded with nausea. He had not gotten "sick" but just didn't feel well.

I had returned to my bed, and he soon after came into my room and said, "Mom, my side still hurts." I looked at him and asked if he was still nauseated, and he replied, "Yes, I have been." Then he continued, "I couldn't sleep well again last night, but when I lay back down, it felt better for a while. Then the pain came back, and I had to take some more ibuprofen."

He was also very uncomfortable with the feeling as though he had to have a bowel movement. This had been occurring for a couple of days, leading me to think he must have been constipated. I asked him to step closer to my bed. I felt his forehead, as Moms do, to check for fever. Then I put my hand on Kyle's stomach, where he seemed to be in the most pain. It was very near where one's appendix is located.

Feeling his stomach, I was very stunned when my hand rested on a very hard spot! I nearly jumped out of my bed, as I was so alarmed to feel his stomach was so hard. "Does that hurt?" I asked. He replied, "No, but don't push on it anymore, please." I was worried about an obstruction or his appendix bursting, but he had not had a fever, and after all I am not a doctor, so I really didn't know what to think. I told him he would be staying home again today, and I would be calling for an appointment as soon as eight arrived.

A 4:30 p.m. appointment was the best we could do, and I felt since he wasn't running a fever it wasn't an emergency, and the nurse seemed to agree. Of course, if his symptoms became worse, we were to go to the emergency room.

I had to go to work and was very uneasy about leaving him alone. Kyle assured me that he would be fine without me. After all, he was thirteen years old. He would phone me if he needed to reach me. So I took Christian with me to the home where I was scheduled to babysit. I phoned my older son, Darren, and asked him if he could keep Christian, age four, while I took Kyle to the doctor. So those arrangements were made. I found myself praying on and on throughout the day and phoning Kyle frequently to make sure he was doing okay by himself at home. I was also making sure that his symptoms weren't increasing and becoming worse. When I arrived home to pick him up, he said he was actually feeling somewhat better.

We arrived at the doctor's office a little early, and they directed us back to the examination room. Our family doctor had a full schedule, so we had to see another physician. She came in rather quickly once we were situated in the examination room. She questioned Kyle about the pain and how it bothered him a couple of weeks ago when he was playing backyard football at his dad's but ibuprofen took care of the pain. The pain did not start up again until he played football again this past weekend.

She began her examination of him, and when he lay down for her to examine his abdomen, she stopped. Her eyes grew wide as she looked at me. Concern was showing in her eyes, and she glanced at me and asked, "Did you know his stomach was so distended?"

I responded, "No, I didn't." I looked at his belly, and it looked almost like a woman's belly at around her fourth month of pregnancy. She continued to feel and push around his lower stomach. Sitting there, stunned at what I was seeing, I was confused and concerned.

She asked me something like, "Didn't you feel how large, hard, and swollen it was?" I responded that I only felt how hard it was on his right side but I hadn't felt the rest of his stomach. The doctor asked me again if I hadn't noticed his stomach or felt how hard it had become. I thought, "How many moms would go around feeling their teenager's belly on a regular basis?" After all, he was my fifth child, and I hadn't ever done that unless they had a problem.

I informed her that I had noticed weight gain, quite significant weight gain over the last month or so. It seemed like his pants were getting too tight on him, and I thought back about my niece Erin's wedding we had attended in South Carolina at the end of December. I had purchased him some new clothes, and when he went to wear the dress slacks for church just a few days ago, they had gotten too tight.

My thoughts went back to our mini vacation for Erin's wedding, and I remembered how Kyle and Christian had been swimming in the motel pool. I didn't notice his stomach at that time. No one else must have either, as they all saw him swimming on different occasions. He went swimming in the motel pool, the ocean, and at my cousin Dawn's pool in their condominium in Myrtle Beach, South Carolina. As I sat there thinking about all of the times Kyle was swimming, my mind took me back to an evening in which I was showering.

I pray often in the shower, as sometimes that is the only place I get some me time. I heard during one prayer time "to prepare for cancer and diabetes." I shook my head and wondered where did that thought come from. As I finished that thought, I heard it again, "Prepare for cancer and diabetes." I believed at that moment that the Lord was talking to me, and he wanted me to hear.

I had taken my four-year-old to the doctor within a day or so after having those thoughts. His glands were so swollen, and they had been, so I felt he needed to be checked out. He had also developed a fever. The doctor assured me that it was his allergies and that he was also getting an ear infection. I returned to the doctor's office with Christian for an ear recheck about two weeks later. They assured me his swollen glands would go down in size but that it would take time. I had not shared with anyone what I had heard the Lord say to me that day in the shower. I made the conscious decision to trust the doctor but knew I would keep a close eye on Christian for any changes to present.

I had also noticed that Kyle was beginning to sleep more and crave sweets. I was concerned about his obvious weight gain but thought I could wait until after our trip to South Carolina and perhaps even wait until the break between Kyle's first and second semester of eighth grade. I brought my thoughts back to the present, and as I sat there watching the doctor continue to examine Kyle, my heart sank. What was wrong with my son? Why didn't I check things out back in November or even December? Why did I feel I could wait to have him examined for his weight gain and sleepiness?

Kyle had been very quiet during this examination and even when all the questions were being asked. He just cooperated and did as he was asked, all the while looking at me as often as he could with those beautiful blue eyes.

The doctor was ready to check his private area, and I said I would be excused during this part. No thirteen-year-old boy wants his mom in the room for that part of the exam. I sat on a stool just outside the door, and a few minutes later, the doctor exited the room and said she would be back in a moment. The nurse told me that the doctor wanted a second opinion about Kyle's abdomen and I was to wait out there for a few more minutes. I waited for the doctor to return with her colleagues and watched as they entered and then exited the room. They gently smiled at me, but I could see in their faces great concern. A gut-wrenching feeling swept over my body, and my heart was pounding out of my chest, ringing in my ears.

"Don't panic. Wait until you hear what they have to say," is all I remember thinking.

Within just a few minutes following the other doctors leaving the room, his physician and the physician's assistant, Tracy, asked me to step into another examination room. My heart was pounding out of my chest, and my heart was up in my throat. I had such a feeling of fear coming over my mind. This wasn't good, and then I said, "Help me, Jesus." A calm feeling crept into my being, not that I was calm, but I could focus and prepare to hear what they had to say with clarity I did not possess a few minutes earlier.

I knew Tracy, as she was a high school friend of my second daughter, Gina, and I thought it was very nice to have someone there that I "knew." I realized she was there as a professional, but I believed she was there also as a family friend. Tracy had been around Kyle when she came to our home to visit Gina during her teen years. I felt some comfort in knowing that she knew us personally.

The doctor said something like, "It appears your son has a large tumor in his abdomen. We need to get him into the CT area of the hospital as soon as we can. We are having an emergency scan scheduled as we speak."

My mind was going in a hundred directions.

"We believe it is cancer."

Panic, disbelief, shock all came swarming into my being. I know my heart was beating out of my chest. I kept asking myself, "How can this be?" I needed to talk to someone; I asked God to help me. No, I screamed within my being for God to help me! I could hear their words, but it didn't seem real.

She was very to the point. "We need to tell Kyle, and I need to know how he will react."

I remember just looking at her. "What do I need to tell him?" I asked.

She responded with she would be the one to tell him, but I needed to tell her how he was going to react to the news. I must have looked confused because she said, "If he is going to become violent, we need to have security here."

Tears were blurring my vision. My son…cancer…violent? I looked her in the eyes and said, "No, he will probably be very quiet and then cry." I then said I needed to call someone. Well, I tried to phone my pastor, Jim Payne, but I had no signal on the second story of the doctor's office building. I needed a man of God. I needed prayer. I needed help to get through the next few minutes. The next few minutes were some of the hardest minutes of my life. Little did I know I would encounter several more minutes that would just become harder as time went on.

I remember the doctor returning to the room I was in. She informed me that we needed to tell Kyle. They were ready for him in the radiation department to begin his preparation for his CT scan. I walked into the room, and there Kyle was sitting, waiting patiently for my return. Fortunately, the nurse, Rhonda, had been sitting with him talking and keeping him company, so he hadn't been in the room by himself for the past several minutes. He looked up at me, and he knew something was wrong. I placed my arm around him, so he could lean on me for support if he desired to. I looked into those beautiful blue eyes as he turned even more toward me.

The physician told him that he had a very large tumor and that it was more than likely cancer. I just looked at Kyle, and he looked at me. My eyes were misty and blurry. A small tear slid from his eye, then quickly more tears began to flow from both of ours. I cradled him in my arms as I knelt down beside him. Those beautiful eyes just looked at me, and I assured him that it was going to be okay. We would do all that we needed to do, and most importantly, God was with us.

We didn't really have time to digest the news as a nurse came into the room stating that we needed to get over to the hospital. I explained to him that he was to have a test that would help determine just how large the tumor was and that they discovered a second tumor on his liver during their examination.

As we were about to leave the examination room area, our family doctor came into the section of the physician's examination rooms. She expressed in a caring manner, "These are my patients." She hugged me and reassured me that they would do all they could to help us discover what was truly going on with Kyle. She was so thoughtful and kind. It was exactly what I needed at that very moment. Her eyes said it all; she was concerned, sad, and very caring.

They kept telling me how we needed to hurry up, but I needed to stop the insanity I was feeling and going through. So much had just transpired in less than half of an hour. I felt like things were spinning out of control. I needed to stop and stand still for a moment. I needed to pause and ask the Lord for help. My opportunity came when Kyle shared that he needed to use the restroom.

We left the office, and just outside the door, he found the restroom. I, in turn, found some coins and used the pay phone. Yes, thankfully, there was one in the hallway! I was able to reach our pastor, Jim Payne. I explained to him what I had learned, and he repeated a couple of times, "Are they sure it's cancer?" I told him again, what they said, that it was more than likely cancer. He prayed with me and said he would see me at the hospital in a little while. I felt a peace come over me. It was a peace that only the Lord provides.

We were sent over to the radiology department of MidMichigan Medical Center, which was just a short distance from the doctor's office. The radiation department of the hospital was literally just across the parking lot. Kyle was given the CT contrast solution and began drinking with much reservation! It was awful, awful, awful! My heart ached for Kyle. I knew from experience that the liquid substance was not very tasty. It was necessary for him to drink the liquid before the IV dye and scan could be performed. Each swallow, or actually sip, he took was difficult, as he was not hungry or thirsty. The awful faces he made were indicators of the disgusting taste he was enduring with each swallow. He found himself going into the restroom several times, not sure if he had to throw up or have a bowel movement, yet neither happened.

I realized during this time that Kyle had been having trouble over the past few days with his stomach. Just the night before, when we were out shopping with Darren, Kyle made several trips to the restroom while we were in one of our local stores. He was frustrated because he felt as though he needed to have a bowel movement but couldn't. Now, here he was once again, feeling as though he needed to use the restroom, but could not go to the bathroom.

I was soon able to contact Kyle's father, Fred, my sister Debbie, my son Darren, different pastors from our church, and eventually we had quite a group sitting with us while Kyle suffered through the drinking of his CT solution. He was full of humor between swallows, and he kept us all in a good frame of mind during this process.

They could not get the IV inserted into his arm. After several picks, pokes, tears, and more tears, a technician said, "Let's try the other arm." Then a nurse, Tami, came to the rescue! Finally, after one attempt, the IV was attached to his arm, and the CT could now be performed. They said they would know soon, but more than likely in the morning, just what the results revealed. Tami had suggested we ask for a nurse to place his IV in the future as his veins were deep within his arm—a suggestion I placed in the back of my memory!

Leaving the hospital, I had to go through a four-way stop, and Kyle and I were talking. I glanced over at him with such love in my heart. I remember traveling the next stretch of the road so well, as it was right in front of the cemetery where my grandma Cox was buried. He said he understood he could die from this. He then said, "You know, Mom, I always thought if I got cancer I'd be old and frail. But that wouldn't be so good either 'cause then I couldn't fight it. So now I'm young and strong, so I can fight it." I looked at him with tears streaming down my face. I was so proud of him. He had a courage I couldn't even fathom. He looked at me and smiled. "Remember, Mom, God is in control. That's what you always tell me."

Yes, I remember, but deep in the inner depths of my gut I was screaming! "God, you are in control, but I feel so out of control. I need you now more than I ever have in my entire life. Show me you are here!" Amazingly, that was exactly when my son reached over and touched my hand. A calm spirit filled my soul at that moment.

*****

My thoughts and feelings were all over the place. How did I feel when I heard the words "He has a large tumor. Didn't you notice it?" I couldn't even feel. I stood outside the examination room, and I couldn't even feel; it was as though I were numb. I kept thinking how I failed to notice his stomach, that it was enlarged, that it was hard, that there was something wrong. I sat on that stool as they examined him. I watched the faces of the other doctors that had been asked to come in and examine him. Why didn't they let me in the room then? Why did they keep me out of the room? They were examining his stomach, not his private area. What was the purpose for keeping me out of the room? I watched as the extra doctors walked out of the room. They looked at me and gave that halfhearted smile. Then the physician and Tracy exited the room and asked me to follow them into another room. The nurse offered to stay with Kyle.

I know I kept biting my lip as I was waiting and breathing deeply. I found myself praying, maybe more like asking, "What is going on? Why are they calling other doctors into the room? Why do I have to sit out here?"

I know I was panicked inside. Fear, worry, concern had to have shown in my eyes as I continued to bite the inner part of my lower lip and kept thinking, "Keep it together, Becky, keep it together." Everything seemed so rushed. People staring at me, decisions needing to be made *now*! I remember wanting a human to talk to, but they were pushing me so hard, so quickly, to make decisions. God was with me; He was there. My son was sitting in a room. Would he get angry? they had asked. No. As I had predicted he would cry. My heart ached, as the tear slipped down his cheek as he watched my face. I had to hide my tears, welling up in my eyes. Kyle was relying on me to guide him into the future. So much had happened in this short time. I had taken the time to phone my pastor once I found a payphone.

Upon arrival at the CT area, I found myself sitting with a group of people. I should have felt like I was a part of them, but I had never felt alone in my entire life as I did during this time. I kept thinking why hadn't I notice this large tumor. How could Kyle not have felt this big hard bump in his stomach? I wanted to cry; I couldn't cry. I wanted to scream; I couldn't scream! I felt like I was in a fog, yet my eyes were not clouded; I could see clearly. My stomach was in a knot. I wanted to run but had to sit and wait. Wait for the next steps, just plain wait.

How does one process that your son has some type of cancer and just went in for his CT scan while sitting next to my older son and his wife as we waited to go in for a scheduled pregnancy ultrasound just down the hall from where we were sitting? I walked with them to hear the results that sadly the baby didn't have a heartbeat. I stepped out of the room. I was so saddened. There was not going to be a new grandbaby to hold, my first grandchild, in my near future. As I looked up and entered the waiting room, I was greeted by a technician who told me I'd probably receive a call this evening yet to schedule a biopsy appointment for Kyle for the next day. They hoped the biopsy would help determine just what type of cancer Kyle had. So I will say again, how does one process this information? I'm not sure how I did it, but I remember turning to God with just one word, "Help," and then I cried out in my mind, "I need your strength!" I couldn't comprehend it all. It seemed so unreal.

Many, many years ago, I decided I would not lie to my children. I share with them age appropriately what is going on in our lives. I knew I would have to answer questions or ask questions that would be very difficult. After the initial visit and CT scan, I had my first hard question, of several, that night. I distinctly remember asking Kyle in the quiet of our van, as we drove past the cemetery where my grandma Cox is buried, what he was thinking. He hadn't said much up to that point about it, but then there hadn't been any time to really talk. He shared his opinion and strength he possessed, and we went about our evening. It was then that he said, "I thought if I got cancer, I'd be old. But now that I have cancer, I am young and can fight it." It was then that I began my life verse: God has a plan and He is in *control*!

The tears would come as I lay in the tub. I soon found this to be a ritual I did on our journey—the safety of my tub, the quietness of the moment, and God's presence to hold me as I needed him to do. I sometimes could sob uncontrollably, but I usually tried not to do this if the boys were awake. I remember saying, "God I don't understand, but you tell us not to lean on our own understanding, but in all our ways we are to acknowledge you, and you will direct our paths." Once again, a gentle reminder comforted me, "God is in control."

CHAPTER 3

That evening of January 26, 2006, I received a phone call from the doctor's office. It had been confirmed that a large tumor was in his lower abdomen and also one on his liver. She said the hospital would be calling me in the morning to schedule a biopsy to help determine just what type of cancer my son had.

The phone rang, and I answered it. I glanced at the clock. It was 7:00 a.m. The doctor said the biopsy was scheduled at 8:30 a.m. and asked if it would be possible for us to make it by then. I quickly responded that we could be there as they requested. I woke Kyle up and Christian, my four-year-old, so we could get up and around as needed. The phone rang again, a voice asking if we could be to the hospital by 7:30 a.m.! Of course, we could. We really did not have a choice in the matter. Did we?

Upon arriving for the biopsy, we found ourselves in the same testing area we had spent so much time in the night before. I learned that Kyle had to have another IV placed, but this time I knew who to ask for—Tami! I prayed she was present, and she was! She accomplished in one try what had taken several tries the night before. The doctor felt the biopsy would be done through the abdomen since the tumor was so large, but we soon learned that they would be going through the liver. Kyle was given some sleep medication to help him relax and remain still for the procedure. During the waiting process, Kyle joked and laughed with us. It seemed to relax him as well as all of those around him. He was taken into the CT scanner, and they were able to get a needle aspiration, which was necessary to determine the type of cancer my son had.

The procedure went well, and they successfully removed what they needed to send on to the lab. We had to wait for the bleeding to stop, which involved four to five hours of Kyle lying and remaining on his side. Oh goodness, how were we going to pass the time?

Humor and cards seemed to be a good way to do just that. Kyle was still under the influence of the medication, and his older brother Darren, who had come to keep him company, was also taking some pain pills for a very bad back. So between the two of them, we had lots of laugher as we listened to their slurs and playful banter. The deck of cards came out, and they tried to get into a good card game and also some card tricks. As we sat there, I couldn't help but think that the results of the biopsy would be known today. Perhaps they may even be known before we left the hospital. I kept thinking, "Lord, what do you have in store for our lives? What path does Kyle have to go down? How am I to walk this path, no, this journey, with my son?"

I remember walking around the hospital waiting area in this section of the hospital. A fast-food sandwich was brought to me, which I ate out of Kyle's view. He was not allowed to eat anything yet, so I didn't want to entice him. We also didn't know what they had planned for him, so we waited. Tami, the nurse who was in charge of Kyle, was a very aggressive advocate for us during this time frame. The results would be known about 2:00 p.m., and we would learn exactly what was going on with Kyle's body.

I was directed into a private room for the nurses in this unit. Within minutes, a phone call came through for us; it was our family physician. My heart was pounding so strongly I could feel it in my temples and chest, plus my legs were shaking.

"Kyle has cancer."

It was now confirmed. The words just stuck there; it didn't seem real. The biopsy gave a "positive" result: my son, aged thirteen, had cancer.

Tami had been very adamant about reaching our family doctor. She knew she was in her office but felt we needed to hear today what the results were. It was Friday afternoon, and she didn't feel it was in our best interest to wait until Monday to hear from the doctor about the results. I was so grateful for her tenacity. She went above and beyond her normal nursing duties. She was very caring and kind. She stayed very close during my phone conversation yet gave me the space I needed to hear what the doctor was about to say.

"Kyle has cancer." The words just stung my ears, my heart, as I continued to listen to the doctor. "They think it is a type called neuroblastoma. It is not one of the better types of cancer, but we have had children come through this. He is also older than the 'normal' age range for this type of cancer. The patients that usually have this type of cancer are around two or three years of age. We plan on sending you down to the C. S. Mott Children's Hospital in Ann Arbor. You will need to report to the seventh floor at noon tomorrow."

"Tomorrow!" I gasped.

Oh my goodness! My heart racing, my head spinning, I managed to jot down the information on a piece of paper that I motioned to Tami I needed. I repeated the information to the doctor and thanked her for all she had done. I looked at Tami, who had tears in her eyes, and truthfully, I couldn't recall if I had tears at this point yet. Shock just worked its way through my body. How would I tell Kyle and my five other children who ranged four to twenty-nine years of age? I sat still for a moment and prayed, "Lord, help me. I don't know what to do or say. Lord, please be with me." Tami hugged me, which I was grateful for. I felt so alone, and yet I knew I wasn't.

I walked across the hallway and told Kyle I had to talk to him in private. He was sitting in a wheelchair, and several family members were seated near him as I approached him. I believe they could tell by my face that it wasn't good news. Tami helped by pushing him into the room, with Fred following close behind. As I told Kyle, I know my cheeks became moist with tears, as did his. He questioned if they had a cure for it, and he was reassured that they had had children survive this type of cancer. He cried for a few minutes and then said with a new strength in his voice that I'm not sure where it came from, "well, we need to do what we need to do." I left Fred and Kyle sitting in the room and crossed the aisle to talk with our family members. I needed to share the findings and explain how we were expected to be in Ann Arbor by noon the next day.

I had composed myself before I approached them. Tears welled up in my eyes but not like it did in everyone else's. Darren, Debbie, Anneliese, stepmother Penny, and some of my cousins were among those waiting for Kyle when he was pushed out of the small office and into the hallway, ready to escape the day's events. I had asked everyone to gain composure before he came out, and they all did. Kyle looked at everyone and smiled. Yes, Kyle had smiled. We wheeled him out of the hospital, ready to begin the biggest journey of our lifetimes, a journey we lovingly began calling Kyle's cancer journey.

*****

As I lay in bed just a little over twenty-four hours since Kyle's CT scan, my mind reeled back to the previous day.

I thought about how the doctor looked at me and asked, "Did you not notice his stomach was so distended?" I had said no. Then she had said, "Couldn't you feel it?" I thought to myself, and probably said aloud, "I usually don't feel my thirteen-year-old son's stomach unless he complains of pain such as he did earlier in the day."

I couldn't believe she was asking such a question. I felt like screaming to the doctor, "My son is nearly fourteen years old—I don't dress him, I don't bathe him. Why would I be feeling his belly?"

I saw him swimming in an outside pool just over the New Year, so did several others family members. Not one of us saw anything unusual. He had gained weight, but it appeared to be an allover weight gain. He was wearing his swim shorts from the summer. I had no reason to suspect anything. Even while wrestling with his little brother, Kyle was never in any apparent pain when Christian was on his belly or back as they tumbled all over the living room floor.

No, I did not know his stomach was so distended! I have had that question and response go through my head numerous times. I've felt guilty over that comment numerous times, and I've cried because of that comment and held myself responsible numerous times over that question and subsequent comments—and the journey was just beginning. How could I have not noticed?

CHAPTER 4

Walking onto 7 Mott for the first time was a very unique experience. It was Saturday about noon. I remember our entourage walking off the elevator and then entering the corridor with its glass-tunnel-like feels. I remember feeling like I was in the movie *Monsters, Inc.*, the part where they are walking into work. I had the feeling of "Here we are, ready to face whatever life is going to hand us." The strength I felt was not from me but from the Lord.

We continued down the corridor. We approached the hall where the rooms began and a Nerf bullet came whizzing past us, then another. Children were laughing and running around. Some of them were pulling IV poles as they went; others were just scampering around trying to find a place to hide. Welcome to 7 Mott, University of Michigan, Ann Arbor.

The laughter and activity w not what I expected, but they were welcomed sights and sounds. Children of all ages were participating in the fun. Their little bald heads, pale and yellowish skin color, and happy, smiling faces bring joy to my heart when I think of that first day on the oncology/hematology floor. Kyle was smiling.

We were greeted by a nurse, whom we would come to know and love, Marnie. She took us to Kyle's room and made sure we were comfortable. It was a nice large room—thank goodness since we had so many who came down with us that day. Let me see. I believe there were about six, maybe seven, of us who came down for this initial visit. We had no idea what to expect. Cancer, my son had cancer. Nothing in life prepares one for a day such as this one. Little did I know that there would be so many days that I could never prepare for as we walked this cancer journey.

Kyle brought with us his PS2, the little portable television we used for traveling, his Game Boy Advance, his iPod, and all the goodies that went with all of them. We brought clothes, not knowing how long he would be staying. We must have looked like we were moving in for a long visit. Later we learned we would spend more time in the hospital than out of it! Oops, I am getting ahead of myself here.

The first thing that took getting used to was remembering that U of M is a teaching hospital. That in and of itself meant there were more doctors than other hospitals, questions were repeated numerous times, and we were told different things by different levels of staff. I quickly realized the beginning of a journey had everyone searching for the right path to follow, and Kyle's cancer proved this theory to be very true.

Liz was another nurse we met that first day, and she was Kyle's primary nurse during this visit. She had the sweetest disposition and kindest heart, as we learned most of the nurses did on 7 Mott. It takes special people to help these very ill children and come in with a smile on their face each and every time they get called into the room. She immediately made us feel at home, and from Marnie and Liz, we learned a lot that first afternoon about how things work on 7 Mott, which I always switch around and call "Mott 7."

Since our visit began on a Saturday, we weren't sure just how much would be done right away. The big question was what type of cancer did he have. MidMichigan Regional Medical Center had done a biopsy of the liver to help determine the exact type of cancer we were dealing with. They said they thought it presented as neuroblastoma, but he was technically too old for this type of cancer.

Well, apparently, MidMichigan Regional Medical Center was incorrect. It so happened that a young man of Kyle's age, named Michael, had been diagnosed with this form of cancer and had been treated at U of M. So I quickly learned cancer knows no age but can come in any form and will try to destroy the life of that individual. Michael did die from the neuroblastoma at the age of fourteen. U of M staff assured us that they would be running tests to make certain of the exact type of cancer Kyle had; if it were neuroblastoma, we would deal with it as we needed.

Blood work, blood work, blood work. Ouch, ouch, ouch! Kyle's veins were not good for drawing blood from. He had really deep-set veins. He cried at times because they would have to poke and wiggle the needle around so many times. He felt like they were digging and digging and going deeper and deeper into his arm.

Kyle cried and cried but always sat very still while the technicians were poking and twisting the needle in his arm. He would just look up at me, and I would say, "Pray," as he squeezed my hand at the same time. He would watch my face from that day forward every time we had to have a procedure or conversation with the medical staff. Early on, it was decided that Kyle would do as the medical people asked, and I took care of all the medical questions, decisions, and consultations. He said, "Mom, I'll do what they ask. You learn what they want me to do." He also shared, "Mom, I watch your eyes. They tell me what I need to know. You know, I wouldn't have cried when they told me they thought I had cancer if you hadn't." I smiled and said, "I know, honey," as I hugged him.

I think I'd like to repeat this lesson that I learned from Kyle. "Mom, I watch your eyes. They tell me what I need to know. I wouldn't have cried that day you told me they thought I had cancer, but you had tears, and that's why I did." Our children watch our faces very closely. Some do not ever share that with us, but my son did that day, and I soon learned that he would watch my face very closely for the journey we were embarking on.

CHAPTER 5

As I sat in Kyle's first hospital room on 7 Mott, I had time to stop and feel. It was January 28, 2006. I hadn't realized just how numb I had felt for the past three days. I found myself purposefully talking to God a lot. I found myself talking with Him more for direction rather than questioning Him why or how did this happen. I sought wisdom to know whom to trust and what steps to follow and the desire for a leading in the direction I needed to take for the moment. After all, He had talked to me one November 2005 morning, saying, "Prepare for diabetes and cancer." I remember thinking why did that thought just come into my mind.

As I was praying this time, I was nudged, hearing once again, "Prepare." One can't prepare for cancer, especially when it is their child who was diagnosed. What did God mean with "prepare"? Well, I would later learn just what that would mean.

But for the moment, I was sitting in a dark room in the early morning hours while Kyle and others were sleeping. I was waiting for the doctors to come in and tell me what they had found out. I told myself, "Surely by now they should know what they were going to do with this probable diagnosis of neuroblastoma."

As I continued to sit and look around the dark room, with the lights from the hallway streaming in through the blinds, I thought about the past couple of days. I recalled how brave Kyle was when I wheeled him out of that little office after learning of his "cancer." He had expressed, "I don't want everyone crying." I told him, "They aren't. But if you see tears, it's just that everyone feels so badly that this is happening to you." He joked and teased about getting a free ride because I was pushing him in the wheelchair—a subject that we would talk a great deal about in the future!

The doctors came in, and they decided after reviewing the blood work and the biopsy results from MidMichigan that more exams were necessary. It was determined that they needed to do a bone-marrow biopsy. They needed to see if the cancer was hidden within the bone. Kyle's dad and I had divorced when Kyle was around the age of four. Kyle lived with me and visited his dad regularly. We all had gotten along very well, with Fred telling me often that I was doing a great job raising Kyle. So I was the primary individual handling the medical, emotional, and mental aspects of this journey.

We learned that no matter what type of cancer Kyle had, it was going to be a process. It was going to require a lot of cooperation on both of our behalf. Fred said he wanted to do his part. The first opportunity came with the announcement that the bone-marrow test was going to take place. The hospital staff shared with us that one of us could accompany him during the procedure. I looked at Fred and said, "Well, here is the opportunity for you to start participating." He looked a little pale but said okay. The staff explained the procedure, explaining that Kyle would not be put under all the way but in a twilight state.

It was nerve-wracking for me to stand outside the door while the procedure was going on. It took place in a room right there on 7 Mott, just down the hall from his room. I paced around or chatted with family members as I waited,. Then some of the attending staff came out of the room. One nurse looked at me and motioned it was okay for me to enter the room as the procedure was completed.

I took one look at Fred's face. He was white as a sheet—maybe even whiter! He looked at me and, well, let me just say, I was the one who did all the procedures with Kyle following that experience. I walked across the room and sat next to Kyle, who was lying on his belly and lifting his chest up and trying to roll over. The hospital staff told him to just lay still for a little longer. He looked at me and said, "Hi, Mom." Then he kept asking where his dad was. Well, the twilight medicine was wearing of, and he kept repeating himself. This is a normal occurrence following the use of the medication. Eventually he woke up enough to be taken back to his room.

They had aspirated bone marrow from his hips. It is a hard procedure on teenage boys as their bones are so strong and that the "drilling" of the marrow is more difficult. I was just very thankful that it was a procedure that Kyle did not remember and never had to go through again as his marrow was not infected with the cancer.

*****

Little did I know just how much I would have to sit and help Kyle get through during this cancer process. Really though, he helped me through it just as much, if not more! He was lying there in that hospital bed, where he looked so big yet seemed so small to me. He was my little boy; no, he was becoming a young man, just roughly six weeks from turning fourteen years old. He was wearing his Michigan State attire and made it a point to let all of the U of M staff know just which school his loyalties were with. After all, his sister went to State, and that should be the school of choice. He would chuckle when one of the nurses would tell him just where their loyalties lie too! Laughter—that was what Kyle brought to everyone who came in contact with him! His nickname became Kyle with the Smile.

He looked around the room and felt very happy. His family was there. Even Gina had flown in from Texas wearing her college colors proudly, along with two of her best friends, Amy and Nicole, from our hometown of Midland. Darren usually gave him some grief about wearing his State colors as he was a U of M fan. Anneliese was there waiting with the rest of us to learn just what was going on with their brother. Heather, his eldest sister, had a hard time about being at the hospital. We all understood, and she and Brad cared from their home.

CHAPTER 6

The next couple of days at the hospital were so crazy and busy, yet there was a great deal of time on Sunday where we had nothing to "do." The attending physician wrote a pass for Kyle to go to a movie and dinner with his family. We went to see *The Chronicles of Narnia: The Lion, the Witch and the Wardrobe.*

While sitting and watching the movie, munching on popcorn, and drinking pop, I whispered to Kyle to look at the symbolism all throughout the movie. This was about the life of Christ. "Wow," he said. As we progressed further into the movie, he would tell me, "I see it. I understand it." Sometimes he would just grin at me. I looked at him in wonder. Here was a young man facing a challenge none of us ever think we would face, and all the while, there he sat smiling and enjoying time with his family. Our next stop was Steak 'n Shake, where we laughed and laughed.

Laughter was the key. Laughter brought everything back into perspective, and sometimes laughter made things hurt. But wait, once again I am getting ahead of myself.

*****

January 29, 2006, Sunday, I remember standing outside of Kyle's room. What an emotional roller-coaster ride it had been. Kyle's dad and I had always gotten along. My emotions were so raw at that time, and I had wanted to share with him, but his wife was generally present. I felt intruded upon. This was our son, no one else's. This was our time. It seemed as though my life was no longer mine. Life was unfolding a path, one I wasn't sure I was ready to go down, but I realized had no control.

There were more tests, more doctors, more questions—the same questions being asked and answered over and over again. Finally, Kyle looked at me and said, "Why do they have to ask the same question over and over when sometimes it's just worded a different way?" I explained that we were at a teaching hospital, that he was encountering medical students, residents, fellows, and attending physicians during that hospital visit and they were all part of the team of medical personnel needed to be a part of his case. I added that if we continued to seek treatment there, he would keep on seeing several different doctors and nurses asking the same questions repeatedly. Then Kyle gave me the look, where his eyes looked deep into my soul, saying, "Remember, Mom, you answer the medical. I'll do what I am told."

Finally, they approached us and felt that they had the type of cancer pegged. They were 90 something percent confident it was rhabdomyosarcoma. Okay, so what in the world was that type of cancer? An explanation followed. Then it seemed that the wheels were rolling forward on what to do next. We could surely tell it was a Monday in the hospital because everyone and their brother came in to visit with us. The social worker, the office of admissions, the newest medical staff on rotation for that week were all coming and going all around us. You'd have thought the circus was coming to town and a huge parade was happening in and out of "our" room. You will notice I will interchange Kyle's journey and our journey because that is exactly what it became.

Doctors came in to inform us that they would be making arrangements to place his central line, and one of them said he needed to talk to another professional about possible sperm collection. "Stop right there a minute!" I exclaimed. "What? What about sperm collection?" They explained that the treatment he would be on would destroy the possibility of Kyle having children in the future. Hmmm, well, we wanted to talk to this person ourselves first and then talk to Kyle. Now here is a tricky part. He was not yet fourteen but must make this decision himself. It surely is funny what "laws" there are and the decisions "children" have to make as though they are adults.

So we were informed about the procedures. She explained that he could be given magazines and nude pictures, and my stomach just turned. I understood the reasoning behind it all, but this is my very innocent son she was talking about. My morals just did a flip, and I immediately started to pray, not hearing half of what she was saying. I knew deep within my being Kyle would not want to do this. I spoke with Fred after our meeting, and he said he could not see Kyle wanting to participate in this procedure either.

Fred and I went into Kyle's room and said we needed to talk to him. We wanted to talk to him in private, so we went down the hall to a separate sitting room. Well, he just looked at us. Then he turned as white as a ghost as the three of us walked down the corridor. Closing the door, I began to talk to Kyle, as Fred had decided that I would be the spokesperson. We began to talk about how his sperm would probably not be good in terms of childbearing after his chemo treatments began. I told him they would have to collect specimens and they would freeze them for future use if he desired.

He kept looking and looking at me, kind of like I was crazy. Then he said, "Mom, if God wants me to have children, He will decide that, right?'

I responded, "Yes, Kyle, He will decide that."

"Remember Abraham? He was old, and God had him have a child."

I smiled and said, "Yes, he did."

"No, Mom, I don't want to do this procedure. I want God to decide if I have children. Remember, He is in control."

I heaved a sigh of relief as I hugged him. Kyle looked at his dad and me and quietly commented, "I thought you were talking to me in here to tell me I was going to die."

"Oh no, honey!" I reached over and hugged him and began crying. I could only hold him and cry some more.

Then the atmosphere in the room cleared a bit, and Fred said something like, "If that had been the case, we wouldn't have been looking as good as we did!"

The three of us went back down to his room, and Kyle kept grinning from ear to ear.

This experience tore me apart. I had talked to my pastor in length about my beliefs, about how I had kept Kyle morally pure and why would I want to present him with images he should not see just to collect sperm. I was so glad I took the time to pray and talk with God before I faced my son with this step of his cancer treatments. The idea that all this had to happen was overwhelming. The pressure to talk to him, to get him to make a decision, it all had to be done *now*, and the process needed to start *now*. Now, now, now! Everything was now—right this minute. My head was swirling, and I couldn't think straight.

Tuesday—yes, it's only Tuesday by this time, and the staff felt pretty confident that the type of cancer was rhabdomyosarcoma. They started to talk to us about the protocol and some of the next steps for this cancer journey. The hospital staff decided Kyle would be released from the hospital but would need to stay nearby. This would make it easier for us to respond quickly when they called us to begin treatments. I asked, "Why? What is the urgency?"

Well, they started to say, "We need to jump on this, and we need to do things quickly, and—"

"Stop! Just stop!" I found myself yelling. Well, it felt like I was yelling. My heart was racing extremely fast, pounding out of my chest. My head was reeling with thoughts out of control. A constant, nonstop feeling was overpowering me! The doctor looked at me, and I asked, "Why is everything so urgent now? Do you know the plan of action? Do you know when the test will confirm accurately that he has rhabdomyosarcoma? And do you know when the central line will actually be placed?"

I got an honest answer. "No, we are not sure exactly when we will get these answers."

I looked at the doctor and said, "This has been a whirlwind four days spent here and two days in Midland since the initial doctor visit. I have a four-year-old at home who is missing his mom and big brother." Then I stated very firmly, "We are going home! We can be called and here within two hours if necessary, but I have a feeling it won't be necessary to drive here that quickly. Am I correct?"

The answer was yes, and at that point, I knew I had made the right decision. David was one of the nicest residents we encountered, and he was the one I was talking with about all of this. We talked several times throughout Kyle's journey about my "very strong decision" after that weekend visit. He shared that he was very happy that I had stood up for my thoughts that day. So on January 31, 2007, Tuesday, we walked off 7 Mott with possible answers but still nothing definite. It had been six days since I had initially taken him to the doctor. We awaited answers, but from our home, not at a hospital room.

I remember arriving home and feeling like the world was spinning out of control. I climbed into my tub filled with hot water and cried, something I would often do after hospital visits. It was where I could release my frustrations, fears, joys, and all other emotions without affecting or upsetting anyone around me.

*****

Christian was so excited to see us and was very clingy. Kyle couldn't return to school, as they didn't want him to be exposed to all the germs floating around the school. Since we didn't know when the call would come for us to return to U of M to place the central line and begin treatment, it was just best for him to remain out of school. We had called a couple of his close friends before we went to U of M, as he had wanted to see them and share his diagnosis with them personally. My family members came over, and we all tried to hide the tears. We couldn't help but think of my dad, who had worried and worried about getting cancer. What would he have thought now, knowing his grandson was going to fight the battle of his lifetime? Cancer had struck our family closer than it had in a long time. Kyle's great-grandfather on my mom's side had multiple myeloma, my dad's brother had died from lung cancer, and my dad's youngest sister had survived breast cancer. My mother, Wanda, was frail from her own health issues. She just kept saying to Kyle, "You'll get through this, boy!"

CHAPTER 7

On January 31, nearly a week after he was excused from the hospital, Kyle chose to do one of the bravest things he could have done. He decided to face his eighth-grade classmates and share with them his illness. As he walked into the school, he was greeted by teachers and administration personnel. He came during their lunch hour. That way, all the students would be located in one area. Kids said hi to him and looked at him, as some already heard that he probably had cancer. He took the microphone and proceeded to tell the students that he, in fact, did have cancer. He told them the type they thought he had but also that we had not had a confirmation call about that yet. He joked around saying, "You know you can't catch cancer from me or anyone. I just need to stay away from school so I don't catch anything from any of you!" He was grinning while he spoke, was joking too, but was serious when he needed to be. I was very proud of him and was surprised at how this normally quiet young man was able to stand before the entire eighth-grade class and tell them like it was—*he had cancer.*

He then went over to his usual table and played cards because "Smitty," as he was known to so many at school, was always up for a card game and had a deck of cards with him at all times. He answered questions classmates had and smiled the whole time.

Teachers talked with me, and tears just welled up in their eyes. So many told me what a heartwarming, loving, and smiling young man Kyle was. They also shared how kind he was to everyone and always just how polite he was to those who came into his path of life. They could not believe that he was so open and sharing about his illness. He was so accepting of whatever the future held for him. To have others see this in my son made my heart swell with pride.

*****

We waited and waited. Hmmm, it seemed that waiting and waiting had become and would continue to be something we would become very familiar with during this journey. Then the day came, and we drove to U of M to visit with Dr. Jasty, the oncologist assigned to Kyle's case. She requested to talk to us first and then his central line, a Broviac, was to be placed.

We arrived at the cancer center on Tuesday, February 7, 2006, anticipating the beginning of his treatment. Dr. Jasty explained how they had thought Kyle had rhabdomyosarcoma but had to reexamine since the numbers were not all matching up. She said they were still doing some research.

I felt a lump in my throat. I was trying not to show any alarm, but my heart was breaking. Why didn't they know? It had been over a week, nearly two, since the biopsy was taken.

Then we talked about the treatment plan, and she said it was best to wait until they had final confirmation on a diagnosis. I asked about the central line placement, and she said, "Well, we won't be doing that today, either." I questioned why not, and she explained that the results they would discover would determine the type of central line to be placed. She didn't want him to go through the surgery to place one type of line when a different one might be needed.

"Okay," I thought, "so what was the purpose for this visit?" It was as though she could read my thoughts. She began before I could ask that she felt we needed face-to-face contact after waiting so long to hear something. She assured us that she would be calling in a few days to confirm future procedures and a positive diagnosis.

We drove home about 120 miles one way. I was feeling very uneasy, and questions were reeling in my mind. I had an awful, uneasy feeling about the whole situation. Kyle wondered why they haven't known anything and when was it all going to start. I couldn't answer those questions. I told him we were having a test in patience.

I cried again once I got home to my tub of hot water. I prayed for God's strength to help me take the next steps necessary.

On Wednesday, February 8, 2006, at around dinner time, 6:00 p.m. to be exact, I received a phone call. Dr. Jasty was on the other end. She said that the type of cancer Kyle had had been finally determined and his protocol had been selected. She wondered if it was possible for us to come back to the clinic in the morning as she wanted to talk to us face-to-face. I said we would be there as requested. Before I had an opportunity to really ask any questions, she said that she would see us tomorrow and go over all the information she had for us.

My heart was beating out of my chest. She eluded any questions about what type of cancer. What had they found? Why didn't she tell me over the phone? What was going on? I felt panic, fear, and helplessness engulf my body. I had a hard time standing and focusing but knew I had to keep myself together. I needed to be able to think clearly! I remember closing my eyes and praying, "Lord, help me."

I called a friend that I knew was headed to church and asked him to please tell the pastor to pray for us during the service. I tried not to show any type of fear or anxiety in front of Kyle. None of it made sense to me. I was afraid they were going to tell us that the cancer was just too advanced to even try to treat it. I called my cousin Christine and my sister Debbie to see if they could ride down with us. I phoned Fred, and he said, "But we were just there!" I acknowledged his comment and relayed the message of how the doctor wanted us there in person tomorrow. I paced the kitchen as I talked and tried to keep my emotions under control. I had heard the tiredness in the doctor's voice, recalling how tired she looked when we saw her just the day before. My gut told me it wasn't good; what she had to tell us just wasn't going to be good.

After receiving the phone call from Dr. Jasty and phoning all others, I paced the kitchen floor. My arms were hugging myself. My thoughts were reeling. She just saw us yesterday! The insistence that she wanted to tell us in person about the information she had received kept weighing heavily on my heart. This, in itself, was nearly unbearable for me. I wanted to know what it was, what we were looking at.

I knew in my gut that it wasn't going to be good news. She wanted us in person! I remember the panic that struck me. I couldn't get ahold of the pastor, yet I could feel God was telling me to turn to Him first. So I got that message, but I still wanted a human to come along side me. But God *is* who I needed to call upon in my time of trial. My head was pounding, and my stomach was churning. I needed to call someone; talking helped me. I did feel better knowing I had reached the gentleman from church, and that calmed me down. God is in control, and He has a plan. But the clock wasn't ticking fast enough for me that evening, and soon morning came.

CHAPTER 8

They skipped the weighing and measuring of Kyle since we were just there two days ago. I looked at Fred and expressed how I wanted just the three of us to go back. I asked him if he could he please ask Penny to remain out there with the others while we had the conference with Dr. Jasty. He agreed.

Kyle's name was called. My heart was pounding out of my chest; I could hear it echoing in my ears. My breathing was rapid and shallow. We stood and started toward the examination rooms. I can't even begin to tell you just how I was feeling. I do remember just asking God to be with me, to hold me up. Then Kyle said, "Mom, I will be watching your face." He told me that was how he always knew how bad things really were. And watch my face he did.

I sat on a couch with Dr. Jasty and Fred, and Kyle took the seat across from us. I was sitting slightly angled toward her so I could see her face and really let the words sink in as she spoke. She expressed how grateful she was that we were able to return to the hospital after having just been in the clinic less than forty-eight hours ago. She said she had the results of the biopsy report, and there was a 100 percent match leading to a diagnosis of a very rare form of cancer. *Numb, stunned, questioning* were just a few words to put my emotions into perspective at that moment.

I remember I thought "'Rare,' that is what we were told about the neuroblastoma, then the rhabdomyosarcoma, and now this one is even worse." I asked her that question. She looked at me with very tired eyes and a very serious expression and said, "Yes, this is even rarer than those." It's called desmoplastic small round cell rumor

(DSRCT for short). It is a very rare form of cancer, with distinctive small blue round cell tumors. DSRCT affects only about 18 percent of the population, with 80 percent of that percentage being males who are around the age of fourteen. She then went on to explain that she did not want to tell me what they had discovered over the phone, as she did not want us checking out any information we may have found on the computer. All the information, I later learned, was not very positive about this cancer. In fact, the information was very grave. She said, "It is a cancer that has had survivors, but the numbers are very low."

I swallowed hard, glancing at Kyle, who was staring at me. I looked at his dad, whose face was red, and I kept asking God to keep me thinking straight, to help me keep my composure. I was being used as the guide. I asked what the protocol would be, and she gave it to us in an outline. They had been in touch with Dr. Brian Kushner at Sloan Kettering in New York. His work has involved the most research and handling of the DSTCT cases. U of M had not handled a full case of this type of cancer, and most medical professionals we got to know had never even heard of this particular type of cancer either. I asked if we should go to New York for his treatment, and she assured me that they had been working with Dr. Kushner. He had given them the protocol to be used for this type of cancer.

The protocol would involve six rounds of harsh chemo requiring hospital stays with seventy-two-hour infusions. The first three would be given, and then hopefully the tumors would shrink and surgery could take place to remove the remaining tumors. Then during the next three rounds of chemo, Kyle would be prepared for apheresis and collection of his blood stem cells for a stem-cell transplant. Then he would receive radiation—in numbers no facility would ever like to give a patient—that would encompass his entire abdomen and pelvis region. They had a strict schedule and hoped to maintain it if all went well. In the event a second surgery was necessary, they would decide the best time to perform it, depending on how well Kyle's body responded to treatments.

Dr. Jasty looked right at Kyle and said, "If there is ever a time that you say 'I just can't do this anymore' or your parents feel that you cannot endure the treatments any longer or we, as a staff, feel the efforts aren't working, we all have a right to stop the procedure." We all understood what she was saying. I was not sure if Kyle had grasped the true significance, but I did.

The doctor reiterated, "We have had survivors." That struck me as though someone had pierced a sword into my chest. This cancer was a terrible one from the get-go. She did warn us that "if this cancer goes into remission and comes back, it will come back with a vengeance."

She handed us a bunch of paperwork, and then she expressed how it was a good thing that Kyle didn't have his central line placed yet because they needed to place the "big guns" in his chest. It was a central line known as a NeoStar triple lumen catheter. It had three ports with larger lines, so when it came time for the transplant, they would be able to remove the stem cells and replace them quicker through that line. We really didn't know what questions to ask, but I felt we had been given adequate time with the doctor. She expressed that she was going on vacation for a week and that was why she had asked us to return to the clinic. She also knew we had waited long enough to learn exactly the outcome of all the tests. For this I was grateful that we had returned so soon.

We walked out rather stunned and overwhelmed, but I felt a sense of relief. At least now, we knew what we were dealing with, and thank goodness, she didn't tell us over the phone because she was right—the computer was a wealth of information, but very ominous information. We were to return on February 13 to have the NeoStar placement done and begin with chemo as soon thereafter as he could, which was scheduled almost immediately following the surgery.

Our family members were anxiously waiting to hear our news. They were as stunned and relieved as we were.

*****

Kyle was a quiet young man, but he was always thinking. He came up to me while I was doing dishes the day after we were informed of his DSRCT diagnosis. He put his arm around my shoulder, looked at me, and said, "Now it's my turn, Mom. You always ask me questions, so here goes. What are you thinking? How do you feel about this?"

I looked up into those beautiful blue eyes and then at his curly long hair and replied, "I never thought I would have a child with cancer. I must trust God and always, always remember He is in control." I paused for a moment, then said, "It seems that God puts people in my life that I help get to their next level, and then they leave me. It seems I end up all alone." I didn't want my son to leave me. I didn't want God to take him. "I have tried to obey God and help others. Now it's my turn to help you get through this journey we have setting before us. And we will do all they ask us to do to fight this cancer."

He responded, "Mom, you do help others get to their next level. Look at my dad, how you encouraged him to go get his GED. And there are so many others you have helped get to their next level in life." There was a pause, and as he squeezed, my shoulders he said with a huge smile, "And, Mom, your rewards are waiting for you in heaven. God knows all that you do and all those that you have helped. We will fight this together!"

How could I keep my eyes from misting over? Well, I couldn't! I turned and hugged the daylights out of my boy. I realized just how truly blessed I had been.

CHAPTER 9

Tuesday, February 14, we arrived at U of M, and it was time for another IV to be placed for surgery to implant the NeoStar in Kyle's chest. Then the journey was really beginning—the journey to actively fight this rare form of cancer that had infiltrated my son's body. It was a journey no one can really prepare someone for, but with the strength of God and the knowledge and guidance from professionals and other cancer families, we were ready to face whatever had to come next.

Kyle cried as they tried to place the IV in pre-op. Once again, they could not place it very easily. It took a long time, and they finally had to get another special nurse to come in and place it. I hugged him and said, "After today, they should not need to poke you anymore, as they will use your NeoStar to draw blood and do medications." This helped him to relax. The IV was finally placed, and then he was whisked off to surgery.

I was amazed that they had finally placed the central line, and he was immediately taken to 7 Mott to begin his first round of chemo. February 14, 2006, was the official start day. They had to wait for tests to verify that he was hydrated enough and then order up the chemo. Well, let's just say, chemo can start at any time of the day or night! I learned that *waiting* would become a word we became all too familiar with as the journey was underway!

I thought of my mom as we sat there waiting for his central line placement. She had told me several times, "Becky, you need to learn to slow down and sit for a while." Little did she know when she said that comment, I would begin soon thereafter to do just that! I know she never would have wanted it to happen under these circumstances, but it did happen, sort of.

*****

Valentine's Day 2006 found us sitting in a room on 7 Mott, with Kyle having a Valentine card delivered to him by a volunteer. We teased about him having a secret admirer, and as time went on, we soon learned just how many admirers he would actually have. It was a volunteer who had made the Valentine to welcome him to the floor. What a kind gesture, and it made everyone smile while we waited patiently to see how this first round of chemo was going to happen.

I do not care to ride elevators. I do not like that enclosed feeling. Needless to say, the only way up to 7 Mott is via elevators for patients and visitors. So that second visit to the floor left me sitting upstairs more than I probably should have. Well, that is what others seemed to think and express to me. People were telling me I needed to get away from the situation for a while. Too much had happened in such a short amount of time, yet it had seemed like we just learned of the cancer. I didn't want to be far away; even the cafeteria seemed too far at that time. I would think of Kyle and felt if he had to endure this ordeal, I would be with him every step of the way, in every way I could possibly be there for him. He had been so strong and easygoing about everything. We would often pray together. Sometimes he would just give me "that" look, the look that said "Mom, we need to pray," and we would.

Kyle seemed to be handling the chemo fairly well. Little did we know that the effects of the chemo wouldn't start to show up until about twenty-four hours after it started to run through his veins. Watch out, the chemo hit with a bang! He began to get sick, and the antinausea medicines that were helping seemed to just stop doing their job. The nurses offered a different antinausea medication, but nothing seemed to stop his discomfort.

Two days into the cycle, he was throwing up and experiencing diarrhea every hour on the hour. My son was becoming exhausted.

While he was sitting on the toilet, holding on to his IV pole, and I was holding his pink puke pan, he looked up at me and quietly said, "Mom, why me?"

I don't know where the strength came from, but as I looked at that gorgeous face, right into those beautiful deep-blue eyes, with sweat and tears streaming down his face, I answered, "Honey, I don't know. Only God knows, and He is in control."

He smiled at me and said, "I know, Mom," before nausea overtook him again. Sweat continued pouring off of his face as we went to return back to his bed. He was so weak I helped him push his IV pole and carried his puke pan as he slowly crawled into his bed.

Kyle never mentioned it again. Never! He accepted the will of God. Now don't get me wrong. He had moments that weren't good, but he never once asked "Why me?" again. I remember touching his face and trying so very hard not to let a tear drop from my eye. I believed what I said, that "God is in control."

Sickness ravaged his body, and he learned to count down the hours and minutes on the IV pumps for each session. He would announce to me exactly how much longer he had to endure the type of chemo that was made of red stuff, which he referred to as the "big stuff." That's the chemo that had to stay hidden under a brown bag to keep the light from weakening it. They kept pumping it into him, trying to kill those cancer cells that were taking over his body. Of course, in the meantime, he was also watching his good cells die too. He would become so weak, and the dry heaves and the runs would violently tire him out. When it was time to end the chemo after his seventy-two-hour infusions, they would continue to give him fluids because he had become so dehydrated. He received more than one type of chemo during a session, and each one had to run at a different pace and over a different amount of time.

Kyle was allowed to eat anything he desired throughout his treatment. However, after the first day, he didn't eat much. A few crackers here and there had been about the extent of any food intake. One time he was having a rough night when a special needs person came in to take the trash out of his room. Kyle looked at me and began to cry. "Why do they make them do the trash and jobs like that?" Kyle asked me as he cried and cried. He reached for me as I was working my way through his chemo med lines. We had hugged often throughout the last month, but that night, he needed to just cry and cry. He always had a soft heart for others, but I believe he was just taken over the edge. His emotions that had been pent up for the past few weeks had filled to the brim, and he just had to release them with me that night.

I recall sitting in his room with my emotions taking over my thoughts and my inner soul. The gamut of emotions that erupted were fear, wonder, questions, anxiety, sorrow, trust, peace, and a gut-wrenching feeling too difficult to describe. Reality began to set in. Life had changed over the past few weeks—life as I knew it would never be the same again!

In the quiet of Kyle's dark hospital room, I found myself watching my son when I couldn't sleep. I read from my Bible with the light of the hallway shining through the window. I would pray and journal and then be jumping up as soon as Kyle needed a hand to the bathroom. I learned that night how to pray a simple prayer, such as "Help" or "Be with us, Lord."

While I sat there, my thoughts were also of Christian. He was still so little, and it was so sad for me that I had to leave him. I was blessed that he was being cared for by Christine and her family. Christine and her husband already had four children but still graciously took us on as a "mission field." They were ready for my phone call on a moment's notice, and I was so grateful for their kindness and goodness that they showered upon us. It helped that Christian had been staying with Christine for a few hours per week, as I was trying to return to school and get my degree for preschool teaching. All of my schooling stopped that day in January, the day my life changed forever.

*****

My faith walk became stronger during that hospital stay also. I found myself studying scripture. I was in a Beth Moore study called *A Woman's Heart* with my ladies' Bible study group at church. I could not manage to finish with my ladies' group, so I worked on it by myself. Sometimes I found myself just opening my Bible and reading whatever that page held. I kept thinking about the time Kyle put his arm around my shoulders at my kitchen sink. "Mom, what are you thinking?" As each day passed, I realized I was quietly asking myself, "What am I thinking?" The one thought that came into the forefront of my thoughts each day was "God is in control." With all that life had handed me up to that point, I realized that my faith was deepening. For much of my life, I don't feel I had turned to God as much as I should have. But this situation—cancer—was a new, foreign road for me to have to travel through. Cancer is something that I never thought would ever be a part of my life, let alone in the life of my child. God had always been there. I just didn't listen for his soft, sweet voice like I should have over the years. I know I had cried out to him so many times, got upset, even angry, so often when it seemed He wasn't listening or doing anything for me in my life. But this cancer journey was bringing me to my knees in a way I never had before. I was coming to know the Lord on a level new to me—a personal level deeper than I ever dreamed possible. I truly began believing God is in *control*. He has a *plan*.

I couldn't understand how or why, but I did turn myself over to God completely in this cancer journey. I had moments of craziness, literally. I felt like the world was closing in on me, but I found myself praying unceasingly, not always asking for things but thanking Him for so much He had given me and provided for me. I started a second Bible study, which was about women of the Bible. Those women had to endure a great deal, and through them, I learned how much they had relied on the Lord. In turn, I too was learning to rely on the Lord completely.

*****

As I sat in my son's hospital room, I thought of everything God does for us—how He talks to us, how He whispers to us when we make ourselves still enough to hear Him. Sometimes we can't hear Him because we stay too busy to let Him into our thoughts or heart.

Sometimes we have the feeling we are all alone, that God is nowhere near us, but really He's holding us and carrying us so close we forget it's not our power we are walking in but His.

God was carrying me through that first round of chemo. He was carrying Kyle. Actually though, I think Kyle just lay back and said, "Lord, here I am. Do with me as you will." Peace. There was peace in the room even though the IV machine was ticking away or the alarm was beeping from time to time, alerting the nurses to an inclusion in the line. There was peace—a peace that "surpasseth all understanding."

*****

I had some rough moments during the early journey. Fred was present during this first round of chemo, as was his wife, Penny. This proved to be a new hurdle for me. I had to share my son with a woman I did not particularly want to have in my life. There had been an incident that occurred in the past that had put a wedge between us. Fred and I had long since worked it out, but I had to share this intimate time with someone I didn't trust. It was difficult and was adding another avenue of depth to my prayer life. God says we are to love our enemies, and I take that to mean those we don't really get along with. This was one of those moments. I was Kyle's mom; she wasn't. He was the baby I gave birth to—he was my son! Then I would hear God telling me, "Remember he is my son first." I knew it was okay to let others love him, but I realized it wasn't easy.

Earlier in the day, I had left Kyle's room and ventured down to the cafeteria. Then I found myself walking the hospital grounds. What a large complex! I was afraid I would not find my way back to 7 Mott! As I walked, I had hoped that Penny and Fred appreciated that I had stepped out. Fred had always told me what a wonderful job I had done with raising Kyle. I remembered a time when Fred and I were standing at the parking lot after Kyle's fourth-grade parent-teacher conference. He smiled at me and said, "Thank you, Becky, for all you do for Kyle." This was not different, as I would do all I could, all that was in my power to do.

Penny was very helpful. She would run down to the cafeteria and grab Kyle anything he wanted, be it an apple, pretzels, or any food. When my nerves were on edge, it bothered me; but deep down, I knew it was because she cared for Kyle, as we all did. We all wanted to try to make him feel as comfortable as we could.

*****

Finally, the first round of chemo ended, and we headed for home. Kyle was tired and exhausted from the harsh medications that had been running through his veins. He announced that he would like to have Taco Bell on our way home. I shook my head and asked him, "How in the world will your stomach tolerate such spicy food when you had hardly eaten anything for nearly four days?" How dare a mother ask such a question!! As soon as he got the taco in his hands, he was eating it. He might not have finished it all, but he did eat quite a few bites. I later learned that spicy foods were about the only foods that he could really taste especially when his taste buds seemed to have been fried up with the rest of his good cells!

CHAPTER 10

Kyle always managed to smile no matter how down he was feeling. Upon arriving home, he asked if he could sleep in my bed since his bed was the top bunk and he didn't feel like climbing up onto it. I agreed and took up residency on the couch. He slept a great deal. He was just drained from his first round of chemo. People would come over to visit, and he would be polite and visit with them for a bit. Then he would usually excuse himself, so he could go crawl back into bed and fall asleep.

I had no idea what to expect after chemotherapy. They had given us directions to follow. The key instruction was to watch for fever. Kyle wasn't eating the best or drinking, but he wasn't having any sign of fever.

During this time, my mood was very low. I won't use the word *depressed*, but probably some would say that's what I was— depressed. So much had happened in one month—learning the type of cancer my son had and watching him go through all he had physically and emotionally—more than a person's mind can wrap around. I hadn't really cried yet. There hadn't been time to do that. Everything just seemed to run together. The protocol we were given to battle this cancer was a strict one. We needed to keep Kyle as healthy as possible during the whole process of fighting this disease. I had to try to have my mind as renewed as I possibly could. Kyle received some verses that I pondered. They were from Psalm 103:1–5 (KJV).

The words I read were

> Bless the Lord oh my soul and all that is within me, bless his holy name. Bless the Lord oh my soul and forget not all his benefits. Who forgiveth all thine iniquities; who healeth all thy diseases. Who redeemed thy life from destruction who crowneth thee with loving kindness and tender mercies. Who satisfieth thy mouth with good things; so that thy youth is renewed like eagle's wings.

I read and underlined these words. I had no idea why they touched me so, but the section that says "who healeth all thy diseases" reigned strong in my heart. God heals.

I had talked with my pastor several times throughout the last month. I remember the day I received the phone call from Dr. Jasty just a little over twenty-four hours after having just been in clinic, the phone call where she announced they had identified the type of cancer with 100 percent certainty. I remember hanging up the phone and feeling my heart ached. I felt like someone was choking me as I grasped for air. I also remember fighting the tears I had. Pastor wasn't available, as it was Wednesday night and he was preparing for services to begin at seven. I phoned a friend that I knew was headed to church, and fortunately, he had his cell phone with him. I had asked him to share with Pastor my phone call and how the doctor did not want to discuss the findings over the phone. I had felt so all alone then, and he had prayed with me. I cried while we prayed, and later I learned he was fighting tears as he spoke with me. I had known by then the cancer wasn't going to be a "good" kind, as each step had already shown that the disease was getting worse and worse with each test. I reached for my Bible and read in Psalms, a book that calmed me down. I let myself fall into Jesus's hands. I didn't tell Kyle how I was feeling, but I did tell him we had to drive back down to U of M to meet with Dr. Jasty as they had gotten back the lab work they were waiting on. I prayed for strength and guidance.

*****

Kyle's dad and stepmom came over every night to visit with Kyle. I was open to Fred coming over whenever he wished to see Kyle. It was a huge step for me to open my door so freely to my ex-husband and his wife daily. I wanted to have as normal of a life as we possibly could, but this was not normal to have them at my home every day. I needed to spend time with my boys like we did precancer days. Christian was whiny and irritated, not understanding what was happening around him. Our home was a small two-bedroom duplex connected only by a carport to the other duplex. Kyle was always wanting to see his dad, but he was not feeling well most of the time. He was always constipated and in misery. He would often say he was full and did not want to eat much and just really wanted to sleep.

I had to talk to someone about how I was feeling, about Fred and Penny coming over so frequently. I did not want to hurt anyone's feelings. I knew they all loved Kyle and wanted to be there with him, but *how* was I going to keep my home life and sanity during this time of trial? I wanted to feel as normal as I possibly could. I had to try to find some way to hang on to some sense of sanity. I hated that our life was flipped totally upside down. How could I keep landing on my feet? As usual, it was God who would grab my leg just when I was about to flip the wrong way. Always turning to Him helped me refocus!

CHAPTER 11

Kyle could still do some schoolwork, but he could no longer attend school. Within a day or so, I learned why attending school was not going to be possible. In about five days following discharge, Kyle was back on 7 Mott with fever. I was instructed to call if the fever reached 100.5 degrees. After contacting the U of M doctor on call and then Nur, the nurse practitioner, I was instructed to take him to our local hospital emergency room. He was feeling so poorly. He had tried to eat that morning but had thrown it all up. He would just look at me, and it would tear my heart up. I couldn't do anything to help my baby. My sister came and sat with Christian as I proceeded to take Kyle to the emergency room. All the while, I was praying, "Lord, I don't know what to expect. Help me to keep my mind wrapped around what I need to do and how to keep Kyle calm during this storm."

No one warned us that Kyle would more than likely respond this way following the chemotherapy. I wish I had been told something like "Expect Kyle to run a fever and become very ill following his chemo session." Maybe they did, but I surely didn't remember hearing it. I did not feel prepared at all for this next step in the journey. I was feeling totally out of control and again was riding a roller coaster for the second time during this journey!

His fever was 100.4 degrees by the time we entered the hospital, and within a few hours, they were doing a chest X-ray and blood work as ordered by the doctors from U of M. They were looking for an obvious infection. His fever had jumped up to 103.8 degrees, so he was then given IV antibiotics. Since it would take an hour for the medication to run its course, I ran home to pack our bags and get Christian ready to go back to Christine's house. She came and gathered up my little son and gave me a reassuring look that all would be okay. I broke down and cried like I hadn't cried before. I was taken over the edge. Tears that should have been flowing all along finally broke free. I felt like a basket case—no, I was a basket case, alone in my home and scared to death about the circumstances that were surrounding me. God says to count it all joy and be content in our circumstances, giving thanks. I kept repeating these verses in my head. I said, "I can't be thankful for this circumstance," and God reminded me, "Be thankful *in* your circumstances." I started thinking of all I had to be thankful for—a local hospital, family who came to my rescue quickly, the telephone, and God being always with me even when I was physically alone or emotionally alone.

Kyle continued to throw up, and the staff began to worry about seizures since the fever was too high. The nurse who had helped us suggested we go via ambulance down to U of M, where he was to be admitted. I learned quickly that the "big gun" NeoStar was going to be a challenge for the emergency room staff during this emergency room hospital visit. I had been instructed how to flush his lumens, but thankfully, the local visiting nurse association had been coming to do that since we arrived home. The staff did not like having to draw off blood then flush the lumens with the saline and heparin. This was a central line that was not used very often, and the hospital staff was very leery on the proper use. I agreed to have the ambulance, and we rode down to U of M, as it was approaching midnight by the time we arrived. I sat up front with the driver, and thankfully, Kyle slept most of the way down.

We were admitted into 7 Mott, and they gave him Tylenol and ran more blood work. Notice I said we were admitted. I realized more than ever that this journey wasn't just Kyle's journey. It was our journey. He was experiencing the cancer, but it was as if cancer was infiltrating our home, our souls, mine as much as his. This disease takes over lives in so many different ways, but it also takes over families. It destroys individuals, families, and life as we once knew it. Pray—that's all I could do. Kyle was so agreeable, no complaining. He would just look at me with those blue eyes, and we did not need to say a word between us. I remember praying for restored health; a miracle that he would be restored completely was what I truly believed could and would happen.

The nurses kept reassuring me that this fever was a good sign. It meant that the chemo was doing its job; it was killing the cancer. But we needed to remember that in the process, it was killing all the good ones too. He had neutropenia, so we had to wait out the fever. Thus, I learned firsthand what it meant for someone to be admitted with fever and neutropenia, "F & N" as we soon began referring to these hospital stays. Neutropenia is an abnormally low count of a type of white-blood cell. He could not fight off infections and was very susceptible at this stage of the journey to the possibility of becoming very ill.

I saw Kyle lying there, a pillar of quiet strength. He did as he was asked, and when asking for his medications, he always—and I can use the word *always*—added a "please" and "thank you." He was teaching me so much that I believed God was giving more for him to teach me along this journey we were embarking on. Later I learned that my thought was so correct!

February 27, 2006, was the first time Kyle had to receive platelets. He did well, and his blood pressure remained good during and after the procedure. Earlier in the day, he opened a card he had gotten from his brother-in-law, Brad Johnson. It talked about being close to Jesus. I found this to be an open door for us to talk about how Kyle was feeling about having cancer and to just explore his feelings in general. Kyle responded with, "I feel closer to Jesus now." Then after a pause, he finished, "I have to rely on Him for everything now. I had to give myself to Him completely. I pray to Him a lot more now, all the time now."

I could see a peace and calmness in Kyle—an acceptance that I am not sure many have during their battle with cancer. I praised the Lord for this gift Kyle had been given, the gift of assurance that Jesus was walking right there beside him, even at times carrying him through the storm.

CHAPTER 12

Kyle had the most beautiful head of hair, curly and quite long for him! He had just decided to grow it out, and this was a huge step for him since he usually asked to get it cut as soon as he could. Normally if he could pull down the bang area and see it, it was time to cut. But not this school year. I wasn't sure I was ready for this new change. The curls in the front looked just like someone had taken a curling iron to it. I kind of gave him a hard time about it and suggested we cut it, but he had responded no. Then the day came when cancer and chemo were going to rule his life for a while. February 10, 2006, we found ourselves standing in front of Ashman Barbers, posing together while my sister, Debbie, took a picture of us together with his full head of hair, a picture that I cherish greatly today.

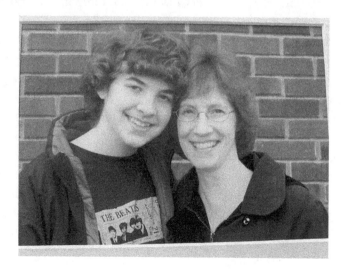

Oh, we had fun shaving his hair! Kyle enjoyed making the most out of every moment he was given. Darren joined us as we entered the barber shop, and the fun began! Darren took the clippers and shaved a strip down Kyle's head. The boys teased each other and laughed as I sat and watched those beautiful curls fall to the floor.

Christian, who was four at the time, went to the toy corner of the shop, sat down, and began to play. When it was time to go, I called his name, and he looked up at me. He broke out into tears when he looked at his brother. "No, I want Kyle's hair back!" he cried out. He was scared of his brother. "I want my Kyle back."

In his loving manner, soft and gentle, Kyle walked over to him and told him, "It's me, little buddy." He took him in his arms.

Christian said, "No, Kyle, I want your hair back!"

Tears gently rolled down my cheeks because I too wanted Kyle's curls back. I had given him such a hard time about letting his hair grow out, and then we didn't have a choice. The chemo was going to kill all the cells necessary to grow that beautiful dark-brown hair. I would question myself over and over again why had I given him such a hard time about his hair. "It's only hair!" I kept yelling in my head. "Hair that my son may never get to grow again." This made me realize how much value we put on things. Why does hair matter so much? Why do we get so upset over the color or the length or the style? It was one of the subjects I would contemplate several times over during the next few months.

Kyle looked very handsome with his five o'clock shadow haircut! He had the most beautifully shaped bald head! You know how some people have oddly shaped heads; well, Kyle's head was a good-shaped melon, as his dad said. I thought, "No, I know God knew Kyle would end up needing to show that bald head of his to the world at this age, at this very stage of his life." He would wear his ball cap, and no one would really notice the lack of hair on his head. His eyebrows were nice and dark and thick, so he just blended right in with the local school swim teams. They were shaving their heads to help gain better speed during their meets. He shaved his head to prepare to run the race of his life, the fight against the very dangerous cancer called desmoplastic small round cell tumor!

Christian had continued to look at Kyle and then hid his face. Kyle had to coax him to come over and sit with him so he could cuddle his little brother and reassure him that he was the same old Kyle he always knew. Eventually, by the end of the evening, Christian had become accepting of Kyle's new "hairstyle."

CHAPTER 13

Kyle's hair had actually grown some between the actual shaving on February 10 and that first fever and neutropenia he had experienced. He was placed in an isolation room with a double-door access to protect him from germs. When a cancer patient is at the f & n stage, their fever can be high and their white blood count very low. Kyle's was less than 1 percent, which meant he had no fighting cells left in his body if he were to get ill. His fever was very high, 102 to 104 degrees, and he was put on intravenous antibiotics. He had wanted the ibuprofen, but he was only allowed Tylenol, as ibuprofen could cause bleeding. His blood was already thinning due to the medications he had to endure during the administration of his chemo.

Kyle was miserable. Just one month after discovery of some type of cancer, while he slept quietly in that isolation room, I noticed hair on his pillow. You see this in the movies, wherein you watch the patient's reaction or see how the loved ones react while standing near the bed. I felt like an outsider watching someone else's life. This wasn't a movie—this was our life, this was my son's hair dotting the white pillowcase on the pediatric floor of a children's hospital. It reminded me of when one gets a haircut and the flyaway pieces of hair stick to their clothing. This wasn't fresh from a haircut, but it meant the chemo was doing its job! His hair was falling out in the front, and his widow's peak was gaining momentum! I wanted to cry. He always found humor in the situation, not a crazy, overbearing humor, but just enough to lighten the load a bit, and that day was no exception! He gently pulled at the hair on his head and showed me he could easily remove fingertips full of hair without feeling a thing. I suggested he not do that as it gave me the creeps! He laughed and then honored my wish.

He was feisty on this month anniversary! The hospital staff tried to get him to get up and move around the room a bit, but he had no desire to do any of that until then. He told Liz, one of his nurses, "Well, if you'd unhook me from this IV, and I could get up and around." Nothing like being spoiled, either! Liz, who had already taken a liking to Kyle, had brought him in some of his favorite Jones Soda to try to encourage him to drink. He ate some Subway and Lay's Baked potato chips and drank some pink lemonade. Then he wanted chili cheese fries. Wow, when his appetite came back, it *came* back. He didn't eat everything but some of each one. I didn't have any more dollar bills, and secretly I was glad because I wasn't sure how his stomach would feel after that particular mixture of food! I said this with a great big smile. What a relief to see him eating and kidding with the nurses and myself. My son was going to pull through this first very hard round of aftereffects from the chemo!

*****

Kyle went through many more rounds of chemo, radiation, and a stem-cell transplant. The journals at the end of this book have more details in them involving those days. It was July 2007. Kyle's sister Anneliese was getting married! We had attended her bridal shower in Port Huron, Michigan, and had chosen to leave from there to head to our vacation south! There was no central line on him, and swimming could happen. We were headed to meet a young lady and her family for the first time in Louisiana before heading on down to Gina's in Texas. Through a phone call inquiring if I was her mom, Jamie and I became friends quickly. Her mom had disappeared many years earlier, and at the time I had the same name as her mom. I was sad to disappoint her, but we were so excited to have this new friendship and we were slated to meet. The *Detroit Free Press* had done an article on our unusual and interesting meeting and friendship. So the boys and I headed south.

CHAPTER 14

I rolled over and pulled the pillow over my head. I still had a couple of hours before we needed to get up and start our day. The boys were going to go swimming at the hotel's pool, and then we were going to be on the road again headed to Round Rock, Texas, to visit Gina. But first we were stopping to meet with Jamie and her family in Louisiana. Jamie is a young woman searching for her mother. Her mother had disappeared when Jamie was twelve years old, and she was yet to be found. My name was also her mom's name, and our birthdates were just a few days apart. Jamie read an article in the *Detroit Free Press*, where I had been interviewed about another patient on 7 Mott. She began investigating and eventually found my number. She phoned me on May 17, 2007. The phone call didn't bring the results Jamie had hoped for, but it did bring a friendship we had maintained to this very day.

I realized Kyle had gotten up and gone into the bathroom. The door opened, and as I lay there, I heard this rubbing sound, like someone was moving their hands back in forth smoothing out the sheets. Hmm, I thought Kyle must be having trouble adjusting in his bed. I said, "Kyle, what are you doing?" as I pulled the pillow off from my head to see what he was up to. It was then that I could not believe what I was seeing!

My heart began to race, my breathing became quickened, and I gasped as I threw the covers off of me. I could see Kyle lying backward on the bed, but I could not see his head. I ran to the other side of the bed, calling his name. More than likely, I was probably beginning to yell his name. I realized he was having a seizure, and I immediately held his head in my hands, trying gently to move his head onto the bed. His body continued to shake uncontrollably. I was able to gently lift his shoulders and square him up enough to lift his head and shoulders at the same time. Once he was safely on the bed, I grabbed the hotel phone and asked them to call 911 and get them to us immediately. Christian, in the meantime, awoke when I put the light on. I told him to sit on the opposite side of the bed and hold his little "night-night" bear so he didn't have to see Kyle having his seizure.

Eventually, the active seizure stopped, and Kyle lay there life-less, nonresponsive. Having had a child have an epileptic seizure, I knew what to anticipate, perhaps vomiting and loss of urination. His breathing was the scary part; it was so irregular and shallow. He was nonresponsive. I called my sister and my pastor back in Midland. I requested prayer with the pastor, a prayer so I could have the strength and courage to make clear decisions. I quickly threw some clothes on and had Christian get dressed. This was all within about five minutes.

My mind would not stop racing. "Why is this happening? Has the cancer gone to the brain? Did the chemo affect the nervous sys-tem and his body is just misfiring from that?" He was breathing bet-ter but still not responding as I called his name. His coloring was coming back, but he was not coming around. "Why is this happen-ing? What is wrong? Calm down, Becky, calm down," I kept telling myself. I asked God to please calm my mind. "Why is he having this seizure? He had a clean bill of health at our last visit. His NeoStar had been removed in May. He is on the road to complete recovery." These questions were booming in my head. I did not understand, but I had to keep my thoughts in total control.

The ambulance drivers arrived. They asked questions, and but they could not get him to respond. We were talking when they noticed he was starting to come around. He finally spoke to them and looked around the room very disoriented. His vitals were return-ing to normal as he talked to the ambulance EMT's. They told me that the hospital they wished to transport him to was in Carrollton, Kentucky, just south of where we were. I talked to Kyle, and he seemed to understand what was going on at that point. We hadn't had breakfast or shower, and my five-year-old wondered what was happening with his big brother. Christian was so confused and overwhelmed I couldn't answer his questions. I told him that Kyle was going to be okay and that we were taking him to a hospital.

My head was spinning. I didn't know what was happening, why this was happening, and I needed to stay calm for my sons. I felt like my whole chest was going to cave in. I wanted to cry; I wanted to scream. I couldn't—I needed to be strong. The boys needed me. I needed God. I began to pray as we followed the ambulance, which was going about ninety miles per hour. I refused to travel that fast and drove at a pace I felt comfortable with. God calmed my spirit. "One step at a time. Just take one step at a time," words I kept hearing in my thoughts.

Kyle was already in the emergency room when we arrived. I told them about his cancer and then placed a call to his oncologists. Dr. Kitchen returned my call first. She asked if they were doing a CT scan, and I said yes. He was having that done as I spoke to her. His neck and head were hurting so badly they felt it was necessary. She requested that I phone her as soon as we knew the results. I found some food for Christian from a vending machine, as it was a small community hospital and the cafeteria wasn't open yet. The nurses brought us juice and anything they could find for him so he would be occupied.

Kyle was put back into his room. They said they needed to start him on antiseizure medications, so they began Dilantin and administered it through an IV to get it into his system quickly. Praise the Lord, the IV placement had gone very smoothly. We both had been surprised how easily they had found a good vein!

Leave it to Kyle, as he lay there wiggling his feet, and the nurse came running into the room! She stopped short of the bed and said, "Oh, you scared the daylights out of me! I thought you were having another seizure with those feet of yours wiggling!" Then she explained from her desk she could see into his room and observe him.

He smiled and said very politely, "I'm sorry, it's just me. I like to wiggle my feet!"

She laughed and said, "Well, maybe you should be still while you are in here, so the doctors won't think you are having another seizure! That way you can get out of here faster!" We all giggled, and much of our tension was slowly disappearing with that conversation.

He soon became tired from the medication and started to fall asleep. Dr. Kitchen and I spoke again when I informed her that his brain CT scan had looked normal. So I asked if I should dare continue on to Texas or should I turn around and go back to Michigan and have him seen by them right away. She suggested I ask Kyle what he wanted to do but also encouraged about us continuing our trip to Texas since he was so looking forward to visiting there again. After speaking for quite a few minutes, it was decided that she would make arrangements for him to see a neurologist upon our arrival back in Michigan in three to four weeks, along with his visit to the cancer center, where she or Dr. Jasty would see him. I also shared with her that the blood work completed looked fine. We also learned that his platelets were staying stable, although not up to normal yet. They hadn't fallen either, so that was a positive sign!

I needed desperately to take a shower and to find a few minutes to release some emotions. That was very difficult to do with Christian at my side and sitting near another hospital bed with Kyle. Checkout time at the motel was fast approaching, and I didn't even know what would happen to our belongings. I thought, "Oh no, another motel charge probably posted to my account too." I voiced my concern to the nurse, and she suggested I go back to the motel and ask if I could shower and freshen up a bit. Kyle needed to remain at the hospital for observation for another couple of hours, so I asked if he would be fine if I left him there while I returned to the motel. I didn't want to leave him there alone, but I truly did need to return to the motel. Kyle was comfortable being at the hospital alone, encouraging me to go do what I needed to do. He felt comfortable there and assured me that he was in the best place possible—a hospital!

Christian and I arrived at the motel to a new manager on duty. He had been informed about our morning and had greeted me with such kindness. I explained how things had gone for Kyle and wondered if I could possibly take a shower before gathering our belongings and leaving. It was checkout time, but he said, "By all means, please stay and use the room at no extra charge." A huge sigh of relief encompassed my being, and I felt very blessed at that moment. The motel had some fruit sitting out, so I picked up a banana and gave it to Christian as I had him climb on the bed and watch television while I took my shower.

The stream of water running over my face and body was so refreshing. Before I knew what was happening, I found my own tears blending into the water from the shower head. I cried silently and called out to God, "Sweet Jesus, please comfort us now. Direct our paths and help me to know what to do with your guidance." His calming spirit was once again upon me, and I felt like He was holding me close to His chest. He was holding me as though I were a small child, and I felt so secure in the knowledge of His love. I thought, "This too I will survive, with complete strength, the Lord's strength."

Kyle was released from the hospital with some prescriptions that needed to be filled. He had eaten some and had not shown signs of having another seizure. We found a local drug store and waited for the prescriptions to be filled. Christian played around on the sidewalk as we sat in the car. Kyle looked at me and said he was feeling better but was having a very bad headache. I told him that it was normal but should pass soon. We talked about what we thought must have happened, and both of us said it was probably an after-effect from the chemo used during his treatments. He teased and said, "Yep, it's probably that one that had to be covered with the brown bag all the time—the big nasty one!" I said, "You are probably sooooo right about that," and we laughed.

******

We had a lot of travel time to make up since we were due to arrive in Shreveport, Louisiana, by noon the following day. I wasn't sure just how Kyle would feel as we traveled. His back was hurting him, and his head was still aching. He put his pillow up against the passenger-side window and fell asleep, but never a complaint came from his mouth.

I was so tired, confused, questioning what had happened. I kept replaying the seizure over and over in my mind. How thankful I was that he had made it back to the bed before the seizure occurred. Was it the lights that triggered the seizure? I kept remembering all the questions the doctors had asked when Gina had a seizure back in 1985. Was there another cause I could come up with, one that did not have to do with cancer? I didn't want it to be the cancer. If it was a part of the cancer, I kept thinking, I hope it was from the chemotherapy he had taken those months earlier and nothing more! I had known other cancer children who were suffering side effects from their chemo. "Please let this be just that," I prayed. However, deep within my being, I knew it was something much worse. I had felt things weren't right with Kyle since March, four months earlier.

I sat in the Kroger parking lot as tears streamed down my face. "Why do I have this feeling? Why do I have this terrible feeling in the pit of my stomach? The doctors keep telling us the cancer is gone! The scans are clean! Why then is Kyle not feeling better?" Overall he was doing well following all the treatments that his protocol entailed. The ascites would not subside, and the platelet blood count would not improve without daily platelet transfusions. He was always tired and was beginning to eat more sweets again too. Sweet treats were not something he always asked for during the majority of his treatments.

I phoned one of my "cancer mom" friends, referring to some of the parents I had lovingly became friends with throughout Kyle's hospital stays. Nan answered and immediately asked me what was wrong. She expressed that she could hear it in my voice.

I swallowed hard and said, "I feel something is wrong with Kyle." I found myself having difficulty speaking the words. I told myself, "Breathe, just, breathe." The words came out almost like a whisper, a very crackling whisper. I felt like I was being negative at a time when I was supposed to be so happy and positive. I felt like I was looking for trouble by expressing my feelings out loud to another person. She asked me why I was feeling like I was, what indication was I seeing, but more importantly, what my gut was telling me. She comforted me with words of encouragement, words that helped me realize that I wasn't thinking the worst but being realistic about what

I was observing. Her daughter was one of the children still having side effects from the chemo, so I knew she would understand my concern.

As I type these words, my stomach is tight, my breathing is fast, and I just remember how I felt at that moment. *Scared.* I was scared that I knew deep down that the cancer that they had warned us about that cold day in February 2006, was coming back, and it was going to be back with vengeance. I sat in that parking lot after our conversation and asked God to please continue to give me the strength I needed, to help me remain positive, and to encourage me to take the steps I needed to get through each day praising Him and holding His hand to get through whatever was coming next in our lives. Actually, I realized it would be Him holding my hand because my hand would slip but His never would!

*****

As I drove down the freeway headed toward Texas, the conversation with Nan played over and over in my head. The scans in April were clean, no cancer detected. Kyle was cancer-free now for four months. So why did he have his seizure? His hair wasn't growing very well anymore, either. I knew it would come in differently, but it was so thin and seemed as though it really wasn't growing. Why did I feel things were not right with my son? I prayed that it was because the chemo and all that it had done to his body during the treatments. Or was it the effect from when he had to tolerate those massive doses of radiation he had endured for twenty days? He had received radiation in amounts that no human being should ever have to endure, radiation amounts that even the doctors at U of M had questioned but were assured that this type of cancer required large doses to kill any cells lingering quietly within his body. His blood platelet count had reached 75, so we were to begin Kyle on Celebrex. It had proven to help fight DSRCT in other patients with great success rate in their long-term survival.

The doctor felt we should wait until we returned from Texas to begin the Celebrex for Kyle since it can cause digestion problems and irritation. The doctor felt he could wait to start the medication and that it wouldn't make a difference in his recovery. I didn't want Kyle to be uncomfortable and have to find a bathroom in a hurry on our trip, so I agreed with their decision. On the road I was beginning to have second thoughts. Maybe we should have had him start the medication. Oh well, now was not the time to second-guess ourselves. We would start his new medication when we returned home in a few weeks.

*****

Kyle's job was to find us a motel for the night. He wanted to go swimming, so he watched for one that had a pool on the sign. We were on roads that we were unfamiliar with as we traveled to visit Gina in Texas. We started this particular trip after attending a bridal shower for Anneliese in Port Huron, Michigan. So we changed our normal route and hoped to see new areas of the country, but it also made finding a room a little bit more difficult!

He picked a Super 8 that was newly renovated and, sure enough, had an indoor pool. We registered for our room and found that someone had brought a cat in the room, which the three of us were allergic to. We could smell the urine in the room air-conditioner. So I went to the front desk and asked for a new room. Moving our things from one room to another, Kyle looked at me and said, "Mom, I am so tired." He placed his head on my shoulder and just looked up at me. His frail body was taller than mine now, and his blue eyes were lifeless and dull. I knew the antiseizure medications would make him tired, and having the seizure itself would wear his precious body out. I assured him that he could get a good night's sleep. He thought of his little brother and said, "But not until I go swimming with Christian!"

The pool was in a room separate from the main complex. Upon entering the pool, we noticed lots and lots of gnats. Kyle looked at me and just shook his head. They attempted to swim, but within a few minutes, we all headed back to the room. "Mom, I'm sorry I guess I didn't pick such a good motel after all," he said as he put his arm around my shoulders. I smiled and said, "We had no idea what we were getting ourselves into when we stopped. But we are safe and have a place to lay our heads for the night." Deep down, I wished we had just asked for a refund and drove on to find a new motel, but Kyle was too tired so that was out of the question. He needed his rest.

He fell asleep very quickly. Christian soon followed his brother's lead, but I did not. I sat in the dark and watched my sons sleep. Every move Kyle made found myself jumping to see if he was okay. I remembered when my second daughter, Gina, had had a seizure while traveling many, many years earlier. I did not sleep the first night after she was released from the hospital following her atonic epileptic seizure. I thought, "Here I go again," but I prayed and asked God to give me the rest my body, mind, and soul so desperately needed. I did sleep, but it was a light sleep; I was aware when Kyle moved and especially when he used the bathroom. The night was uneventful, and after breakfast, we were ready to hit the road again. We were off to meet Jamie and her family in Bossier City, Louisiana.

*****

Let's go swimming! That was the first order of business when we arrived at Gina's in Round Rock, Texas, on July 4, 2007. The boys found themselves splashing and laughing and enjoying themselves following our three-day trip. We were at the pool early, before the picnic crowd arrived for the afternoon. We liked to get to the pool around 10:00 a.m. and swim for an hour or so. The pool was all ours to enjoy, and the boys could be silly. Kyle did swim, but he didn't get in and out of the pool like he usually did. He seemed to swim and then get out and just watch Christian from one of the chairs along the side. Kyle was just so happy to be able to swim again. He seemed happy, almost content, to be sitting there with us in the sunshine. His central line had been removed in May, and he just had a peace about him while hanging around by the pool, being able to jump in and out at his discretion.

Fireworks were next on the agenda for this Fourth of July! We went to a public area and watched the fireworks and an outdoor movie while enjoying the typical fair foods. Kyle rode with Gina to the fair, and they came up to me laughing and teasing about something Gina had done while driving. Apparently, several grasshoppers had gotten into the car and were jumping all around inside. She started to do a dance in the car, which required Kyle to step in and help with the steering wheel. By the time they reached us at our seating area, they were laughing and giggling about the whole ordeal. Those eyes of Kyle's were shining with glee as he retold the story play by play to all of us.

Kyle sat and savored the excitement of the fireworks, remembering how the year before he had been in the hospital on that Fourth of July with fever and neutropenia, unable to truly enjoy the spectacular lights that illuminated the evening sky. Oh, he loved firecrackers too. So he purchased some, which were legal in Texas but not in Michigan, and enjoyed setting off a bunch of them with our family present.

Not being a complainer, Kyle kept it quiet that his head was hurting quite a bit again. He wanted to enjoy each moment he could and laugh and joke with those around him. The boys and I had gone to a friend's house, and Gina had picked Kyle up for an outing. As Kyle was walking out to the car, it appeared that he tripped on the edge of the sidewalk. He fell to the ground. I ran toward him, and he said, "Mom, I am fine, just twisted my foot on the sidewalk." He was weaker than usual, but he went off to join his sister with a great, huge smile on his face.

As he was walking toward the car, I took a long, lingering look at him. His legs were so thin—not only his legs but his whole body. His back had hurt most of the night as he was trying to sleep. He could not get comfortable and had not slept much. When I asked him how he was feeling, he had replied, "I'm okay." He always smiled no matter what was going on with him. But I could see deep in those eyes that something was not right. His beautiful blue eyes were sad sometimes, but he kept causing mischief and laughter, his humor continuously showing through.

*****

I looked at that boy of mine and remembered a moment from a few months earlier as he walked to the car to go with Gina. The memory made me smile then. It still does today.

I had made a promise to Kyle that I would never again give him a hard time about growing his hair out. You see, that was a subject we discussed in depth before his cancer discovery. He had let it grown longer than he ever had, and I didn't care how it was curling, even with his bangs looking like a curling iron had curled them up. After the initial cutting in preparation for chemotherapy, I promised him he could wear his hair any way he desired when it grew back. Well, I kind of went against my word, but just a little. His hair had begun to come in by late winter and had grown straight as all get-out, totally opposite of the hair we had cut off a year earlier.

I noticed it had slowed down in its growth and thickness, which had bothered me for a few months. No one else had mentioned it, so I was not sure if anyone else had noticed, but I had. I had the privilege of seeing other children growing their hair back after completing their chemo treatments, and it was coming in quickly and thick. Each patient is different, and their particular treatment varies. So I knew Kyle's hair might not come thick and curly as it had been, but his hair just didn't look healthy to me.

So to help his hair not look so shaggy, I suggested we get it trimmed. He said, "Mom, you said you wouldn't ask me to get a haircut again!"

I said, "I know, but just a trim would make your hair look thicker and neater."

Gina talked to him about it, saying, "Mom is right this time, Kyle." So he agreed to get a trim, and afterward, he was glad we had gotten it trimmed because it looked and felt better.

He got out of the chair and tugged his shorts up as they were falling down, then he plopped his NY hat on his head and placed his dark-orange sunglasses on his face and grinned all the way out of the shop. To celebrate this first haircut, Kyle asked if we could stop at Sonic and got one of their ice cream treats to celebrate. Yum! Going to Sonic was just one of the many treats Kyle enjoyed again since he liked food once more!

*****

Kyle loved the Food Network programs. He had seen the program featuring the Salt Lick, which is located in the Austin area. We had to go eat there! You see, Kyle decided he was going to become a chef. He wanted to try all the eateries he could, although his own taste buds were limited. I would tease him when he asked to go explore a new restaurant if he was going to try something new, and he would say, "We will see, but probably not!" I often asked, "How do you plan on cooking when you won't taste anything new?" and he always said he would figure it out later. But he loved to watch the *Iron Chef*, Alton Brown, and others and vowed that one day he was going to cook just like they did.

I wasn't sure if Kyle was up for dining out, but he assured me he was more than ready! You see, Kyle had not been sleeping well for the past few nights. He would be up in the night moving from the bed to the couch to the chair. He would come to me and ask for more pillows because the pain was so bad and the beds were feeling very hard on his back. He was also getting hot very easily. Other than expressing how it hurt to sleep or lie down, he never really complained. He was so excited to go to the restaurant. Finally, he was going to try the food he had heard so much about on the television shows.

There was a lengthy wait time at the restaurant. We opted to wait outside under the veranda. Kyle tried to sit, but he couldn't find a comfortable position. He walked around, drank some water, and kept mentioning just how hot he was feeling. He tried to lie down with his head on my lap for a bit and then asked to go to the car so he could sit in the comfort of air-conditioning. He walked back to the car and rested as we sat and waited a little while longer for our table. It was our turn to be seated, and I went to the car so he could join us in the restaurant. As we walked into the restaurant, he looked the whole place over, the ovens, the atmosphere, and then he said, "It is so hot in here." He was correct. The section we were in did not have air-conditioning, and the room that did was full. Smoke from the barbecue filled the air; the aroma of cooked brisket and other meats teased our pallets as we waited to order our family-style food. Kyle smiled, but his eyes were so sad. He kept taking his hat off and looking at me with a "Help me, Mom" kind of expression.

He tried to eat but then said in a panicked voice, "I have to get out of here! Why would they put us in a convection oven to have our dinner?" I gave him a questioning look, and he continued, "Well, they have a metal roof, heat inside these brick walls and no fans or air—it's a convection oven! Mom, I need to go back to the car!" and off he went by himself back to the car. He had eaten a few bites, but he was very uncomfortable. I ate and made sure Christian had enough to eat, and then I left him at the table with Gina, her boyfriend, and some other friends who had joined us for our outing.

Upon arriving at the car, I found Kyle lying down in the back seat. He sat up when I opened the door, and as I got into the front seat, he had tears in his eyes. He was so sad. He said, "Mom, all I wanted to do was eat here and enjoy the restaurant." It was so hot; he was sweating and very uncomfortable. I hugged him and asked if he was ready to go home. "No, just back to Gina's but not quite yet." He then got out of the car and asked to walk with me back to be with the others. The sun had begun to set, and he wanted to stand around and talk with everyone.

I couldn't figure out why he was so much hotter than the rest of us. He always was a boy who couldn't tolerate the heat as well, but he had never had this problem before. He looked at me after about ten minutes of talking and laughing with the others and whispered to me that his head hurt and that he was very tired. He asked if we could please leave. We did, and then he asked to stop and get his favorite Amy's ice cream as we came back into downtown Austin. We stopped, but he didn't order any ice cream. He said he would just take a bite of Christian's or mine if I ordered any. He wanted to see downtown and ride through it before we went back north to Round Rock. My heart sank—something was terribly wrong with my son. He couldn't eat, was drinking very little and asking to see the things he enjoyed. "Just one more time," he kept saying. Deep down inside, I knew Kyle was silently telling me this was going to be his last visit to Austin, Texas.

CHAPTER 15

I have a tendency to stay busy when I am bothered or upset. I find myself cleaning or rearranging to work off the excess stress or energy. A rocking chair has always been my best friend. But amazingly I found myself in a hot bath tub most nights following a hospital stay. I am not sure if it was due to the fact of the community shower/bathroom we had to share on the floor of 7 Mott or just the warmth of the water soothing my tired body. I have since discovered just how soothing water in general can be. I would fill the tub as full as I could and escape to the bathroom after Christian was in bed and Kyle was safely snuggled in his blankets on the love seat, watching one of his favorite television shows.

As I relaxed quietly in the tub, I would try to clear my mind. I would just let the thoughts flow easily, and most times, I would commune with God. I would often think about that November morning when I heard, "You need to prepare for cancer and diabetes." I remembered just how I wondered where in the world did that thought come from and then heard it again, "Prepare." The shower was my quiet time with God. I had found that this was the one place of uninterrupted worship and prayer with the Lord I had during my day. The water pouring down over my face and body was just a releasing time for me, relaxing my mind and body, which helped me to focus on the things God wanted me to rather than on things I thought were important.

As the tears would flow, I found great peace with my thoughts focused on God. Knowing he was in control, and He had a plan. I couldn't understand, but I trusted him.

*****

Kyle had a few hospital stays that were a bit lengthy. The ones that lasted for two to three weeks were very difficult for me to find time to be alone with God because Kyle was usually rather ill during these times. I would walk the grounds at U of M when I could leave Kyle's room for short periods of time. I remember especially the times that were not routine just how hard it was to keep my perspective correct! When Kyle had pneumonia due to MRSA (methicillin-resistant staphylococcus aureus) and especially during his last hospital stay, I found my way to my beautiful red van, where I cried and cried. Sometimes I would talk out loud to God. I would cry out to the Lord in my time of need. I would ask him questions. I would ask for answers, guidance, strength, and more. Sometimes I felt like punching the back of the seat but knew that wouldn't do any good. I would just squeeze and hug a pillow or blanket, and there I found His love and gentle tenderness.

When I quieted down, I knew God was holding me in His arms just the way I hold my loved ones ever so closely. I longed for human arms to hold me, but somehow God's arms were circling me, and a peace would just encompass me—a peace I could not explain, a peace that ran deep into my soul. Then I would realize everything was as it should be. I would get exhausted from my release, but it was a healing tiredness. I would feel being refreshed anew, knowing that God was walking with me each step of the journey.

*****

I had to call Kyle's dad and my family members.

I don't remember sleeping much that night. I just wanted the clock to quickly move so we could be on our two-hour car ride to Ann Arbor to hear exactly what was going on and the plan they intended to use to fight this cancer.

*****

As I sat and watched my son become so sick during one f & n, I became very concerned. His fever continued to spike. They couldn't get it under control. They had cultured his three NeoStar line, and nothing had shown up. However, as usual, they had him on an antibiotic. He became so disoriented and delusional that it was scary to watch. He wasn't like the Kyle we all knew who was always talking goofy and out of context. He was very edgy and irritable this time. Liz, his main nurse, was on duty that particular day. She came into the room and said, "I don't know what's up with Kyle, but something is wrong." As it turned out, he had MRSA. The infection was affecting his brain. One of the cultures finally came back positive for a bacterial infection, and he had this terrible staph infection running rampant through his body. They switched up his antibiotic and other medications.

I sat down with the doctors on that day when they told me he had an infection in his lines. I began with few questions and then asked, "Is it MRSA?" The attending physician stopped, looked at me, and asked me why I thought of that. I looked him in the eyes and politely said, "Well, I've overheard that it is a staph infection, and the one I know is MRSA and he is in quarantine now." The doctor proceeded to ask if I was a medical professional, to which I responded no. So he questioned how I knew about MRSA and its characteristics. I kindly and quietly responded, "My dad had MRSA and died from the complications it produced." He stepped a little closer to me and said, "Yes, Kyle has MRSA, but we are getting it under control."

I'm not sure if I was relieved at that point or not. I knew he wasn't doing well, and the antibiotics he had been given for several days weren't doing anything, so now they would get him on the "big guns" and pray that the infection could be stopped. My early thoughts were that perhaps the chemo medications he had been on were causing some neurological issues, but as soon as the new antibiotics were in his system, we saw an improvement. I know my eyes and heart were sad during this time, yet it was during that particular hospital stay that another case of this rare form of cancer came to 7 Mott, and the nurses/doctors had asked if I was willing to encourage this new family in their walk with DSRCT. As I sat in that large hospital room, the suite with lots of windows to see out of, I could only respond, "Of course, I will." I got their name and where I could find them. I prayed and soon thereafter walked into Eugene's room.

I saw the fear, the questions, and the anxiety of this family. I saw a very encouraging and, soon learned, a very faith-filled family. Their faces reminded me of how I felt the day I learned Kyle had DSRCT. I could see the devastation of such an unforgiving cancer, one that rears its ugly head and an unforgiving vengeance and sneaks upon its victim and snatches their lives away quicker than one can even comprehend. We were there to fight this ugly diagnosis of DSRCT together.

As we became acquainted and began to discuss our journeys thus far about this unwelcomed guest in our lives, I learned that unlike Kyle, Eugene had lost a great deal of weight. He had a main tumor in his abdomen, causing loss of appetite and severe weight loss. Having tumors in the abdomen is one characteristic of this specific cancer. Eugene was thirteen, like Kyle, at the time of diagnosis. We exchanged phone numbers and sat and chatted a while longer. This would be the first of the many times we would talk and spend time together, becoming a family of our own.

I remember this hospital stay well and our little roommate at the time. His name was Michael, and he was in with a blood disorder. He was about six years old and a regular visitor to the seventh floor. His parents couldn't visit him regularly; therefore, I stepped up and helped him order his meals and play games with him. It felt very natural for me to help Michael. I love to help others, and children truly do have a special place in my heart. When Kyle was sleeping, Michael helped fill my day with sunshine. It was a little unusual for Kyle to have such a young roommate, but we welcomed Michael with open arms. He was also a "clean" patient, which meant he wasn't sick or contagious, so he could be in the same room with Kyle. He smiled a lot, but he was so quiet, even when he was playing video games or watching TV. He was full of energy and life. Even though he was in for his own reasons, he helped bring smiles to my face.

Kyle was on precautions, which meant the nurses gowned up and wore masks when treating Kyle. I knew MRSA was serious, even deadly. I would sit by his side and would just hold his hand while he slept. I am very thankful that the room we were in for that stay was the suite; otherwise, I would have had a very enclosed feeling during this particular visit. MRSA was, and is, scary. Having watched my father fight the ill effects it had on his body had me concerned for Kyle. Being able to walk to the windows and look out toward the city of Ann Arbor helped ease my nerves. I wrote in my journal and prayed.

Slowly, Kyle responded to the antibiotics and was able to go home. Another battle fought and won and more experience in the medical field of life as a mom to a son with cancer.

CHAPTER 16

There were so many thoughts as I drove and then the reality set in.

The room was dark, except for the wall night lights shining just enough to guide us in the room. Kyle was sound asleep, exhausted from the long three- to four-hour MRI. Yes, it took them what seemed like forever to get him to be still enough to get good images. He was so exhausted from the pain—the pain that stopped him from lying still, the pain that he didn't understand, the pain we didn't understand.

How fast the past couple of days had gone, yet they seemed to drag on. Hadn't I just driven to and from Texas with Kyle and Christian the last couple of days? Kyle came down the stairs in his sister's condo and lost his step as he slightly tumbled down, catching himself. His eyes had looked at me with a fear, a scare, a concern that he couldn't control his own movements as he desired. "Mom, it's time to go home," he had said, with a quiet, sadness. I helped him get up and continue down the stairs. His head was hurting; his legs were weak. Those blue eyes, those sparkling blue eyes were pleading. Without a word, I knew things were not right, something was terribly wrong. We agreed. It was time to pack up and leave the next morning.

Gina went off to Houston, and we headed on to our drive back to Michigan. Just the boys and I were traveling. The van wasn't overpacked, and I had cleared the very back seat out so Kyle could try to lie down. He was in so much pain, as the bones in his back felt like they had stuck out, making him so uncomfortable. We made a bed of pillows to bring more comfort. As we traveled, Kyle would try to get comfortable, moving very slowly from the middle seat to the back.

We came by a famous restaurant in Missouri that Kyle had watched on the Food Network channel. They would throw biscuits/rolls across the room for you to catch, and it appeared to be a fun place to eat. On the way down, we agreed to stop by and try it out. We stopped at a motel very close to this eatery, and I asked Kyle if he wanted to have dinner there. "No, Mom, I'm too tired, and I don't think I could catch the rolls. Let's just go home," he said wearily.

A stop at Burger King just to grab a bite to eat was our mid-day agenda. Kyle opened the side doors, stepped out, and fell to the ground. My heart stopped. I ran to get him with tears in my eyes. I reached down to help him up. Christian stood with a frightened look on his face. He was confused, not knowing why his brother fell. "Mom, it's okay...my legs just fell asleep. I can get up," Kyle said. The determined look on his face caused me to step aside. I didn't want embarrass him, so I stepped back and offered him my hand.

A gentleman had observed the incident from inside the restaurant. He came outside and asked if he could help. Kyle accepted my hand as the man stood by and made sure he didn't lose his balance. We walked in the doors, and Kyle needed to use the restroom. My heart stopped. What if something happened while he was in there? How could I help him, or how would I know? As though the man could read my mind, he quietly said he would go into the restroom and be there if Kyle should need any help. Very kindly and very privately, he assured me that he would give him the privacy he deserved.

As we approached Michigan, I mentioned how I felt we needed to go directly to 7 Mott. Kyle pleadingly looked at me and said he really wanted to just spend one more night in his bed. He just wanted to be in his own bed. Deep down, I heard the "one more night in my bed..."

We arrived home early evening. Kyle made his way to the blue loveseat he loved to sit and lie on. He looked relaxed as he slept; he was at peace. He asked me sometime in the night to climb up on the top bunk bed, his bed. I fought him for a while until I agreed, not knowing if I'd be able to get him down out of bed in the morning.

CHAPTER 17

I phoned my sister and brother-in-law, Debbie and Don, to come over to help get Kyle down out of bed. We managed to get him down, and as he prepared to go to U of M, as we prepared to leave for Ann Arbor, we had no idea what awaited us. I watched my son and knew something was terribly wrong. Something told me that he would not be coming home again, that he'd never sleep in his bed again.

The ride to Ann Arbor was painful for Kyle. We arrived at the emergency room as the doctors had instructed us. They had been waiting for us, so they immediately put us into a room. The medical staff came and examined him, with an MRI already scheduled. It's a rarity to have an MRI done instantly in the emergency room. However, we had been in phone contact with the doctors, and they were well aware of his declining health; therefore, they had it scheduled for as soon as we arrived.

We were able to place him on the MRI table, but he was in so much pain. They administered pain medications as much as they could. They were at the maximum allowable amount they could give without the SWAT team there to oversee the dosing. Kyle could not get comfortable, and before we knew it, a great deal of time had passed by. I discovered it had been literally two and three hours with him lying on the scan table, as we tried to get the different MRI views the doctors had ordered. He had to go to the bathroom, so I had to help him with the portable urinal. He was not embarrassed or ashamed, but he did apologize that he needed my help. I smiled and assured him it was my pleasure to help him as he needed me to.

Then we were having trouble getting him to just lie still even for a few minutes. I finally had to get close to his face and look him square in the eye and say to him. "Kyle, they are trying to see if you have any tumors in your brain. They need you to stay very, very still."

He looked at me with a sorrow, a sadness, saying, "Okay, Mom."

I lovingly gazed at those blue eyes. I prayed with him and moved away once again from the MRI machine. This time, a peace came over him as he lay still to complete the final tests necessary. We were soon released to a room up on Mott 7—our second home.

CHAPTER 18

"Mom, am I past the part where I'm going to die?"
I knew the answer to this question as I sat in the quiet of Kyle's room on Mott 7, listening to his breathing in the wee hours of the morning. He looked so small, although he was 5 feet and 10 inches tall. He had become skin and bones, as we say—no meat to him at all. I didn't need a doctor to tell me what God had laid on my heart back in March. The cancer was back. I knew deep in the pit of my stomach it was *back*.

The hall light streamed into the darkened room, which was only illuminated by the night lights casting enough light to see the eyes, faces, and expressions on the white coats' faces. As they approached me, I looked them in the eyes and saw the news all over their faces. I did not know these two young doctors. The news they were about to give to me had to be hard for them to deliver. Not knowing me might have made it easier, yet how do you tell someone their child is dying? How do you tell someone that someone's cancer has returned with a vengeance?

The Holy Spirit had engulfed me while I was sitting in that recliner rocker. I knew already the news I was to receive even before they walked in. I knew something was wrong way back in March, back to when I was sitting at the Kroger parking lot as I cried and eventually phoned a "cancer mom" I was close to.

I spoke first. "I already know. Kyle's cancer has returned. That there is nothing more we can do. I know my son is dying."

The white coats were stunned. They were almost speechless. I asked some questions, like were there a lot of tumors in his brain, where else did they show up, and how long did they feel he had left with us. They answered as much as they could but kept looking at me and asking if there was anyone they could call for me, if I needed to talk with someone. I assured them I had talked with the one that mattered most—my Lord, that He was with me at this very difficult time, that He was holding me up at that moment. As we walked out of the room, they once again looked into my eyes and said, "Are you sure you don't want us to call someone for you?"

"No, I knew what I need to do and who I need to contact," I said.

Tears were welling in our eyes. Hugs were exchanged. I walked down the hall, hit the elevator up button, and went to the eighth floor. I approached that little chapel I so frequently visited, no different than times before at 2:00 or 3:00 a.m., but this time, I cried out to the Lord for the strength to do as He willed for the next few minutes and days to come.

I proceeded to call family and tell them the news I had received. I had debated on waiting until later in the morning, deciding to make the calls everyone was waiting on right then. I had to tell them that their brother, nephew, and son was dying.

How was I going to tell Kyle, "Son, you are dying"? That, to me, was going to be the most difficult one to tell—the boy who had fought so hard, the boy who smiled in the midst of the fight, the boy who had only questioned once "Why me?" This was the boy who accepted cancer with his head held high and, grabbing the Lord's hand, walked through all the adversity these past eighteen months that cancer and the treatments had placed on him. How was I going to tell him?

Family started arriving later that morning. It was difficult reaching Kyle's dad, as he had gone camping. Thankfully, one of Kyle's cousins and Anneliese had remained close. She was able to reach Jennifer, who let Fred know.

Later that morning, the attending physician came into the room. He was one we had had previously, but not one of the "regular" ones we had gotten to know so well. He was very gentle and caring. Kyle was to begin brain radiation. He could receive up to ten doses, one given per day. There was nothing else they could do.

He showed us the MRI pictures and pointed out all the little small round blue cells that were indicative of desmoplastic small round blue cell tumor cancer. Even I, a nontrained professional, could see them all over his brain. Apparently, the cancer returned in the meningeal lining of his lower spine and in his neck and brain. The cancer returned exactly outside of the area that had received radiation. It was as though the cancer cells had attached themselves to the very next possible cell outside of the full-body radiation area.

"The cancer will come back with a vengeance…if it returns. There is nothing more we can do if that happens. If the cancer comes back, it will be with a vengeance. If…there was no more if…it had returned." My mind was reeling as I looked at this MRI. The original words of Dr. Jasty kept going over and over in my mind. These words were not supposed to become a reality—words that were spoken but weren't going to affect my son. My son was full of cancer again. How much at this time, I had no idea. I just knew it had returned. And we were going to do what we could to help make his final days on earth a little easier if we could.

CHAPTER 19

Kyle was having seizures. The doctors at U of M had felt he was
on a very strong dose of antiseizure medications, so they had
lowered the dose. He had continuous headaches, which the hospital
in Round Rock, Texas, had said were seizures not breaking through
completely. He was so lethargic too.

Anneliese had been with him since the day after we learned he
was dying. I had stayed at the motel with Christian for the night,
returning to U & M in the morning. We were parking the car on
the top floor of the parking garage when my cell phone rang. It was
Anneliese with a very panicked-sounding voice.

"Mom, where are you?"

"Just parked the car. Why?"

"Kyle had a bad seizure. Get here as quickly as you can!"

I took Christian's hand, and we began to run for the stairs,
with several flights to descend. Then we went through the hospital
entrance and up the elevators to the seventh floor on Mott.

When I opened the door, I saw a very scared, white-as-a-ghost
daughter sitting by her brother. She had tears filling her eyes as she
explained to me what had just happened. Kyle had had a rigid seizure.
As she stood him up, he became stiff as a board and was shaking. She
couldn't move him. My nephew Erik was with her and helped get
him back into his bed. He was sleeping when I arrived.

Kyle was in and out of sleep. Hot and cold spells hit his body.
He was aware, but not aware. I would have moments of lucidness
with him, and then he would be hallucinating so badly. I told him
a few times he was dying when he asked why was he in the hospital.

I was with him alone in the room. He opened his eyes. He was very aware of his surroundings. The antiseizure medications seemed to be working again; the staff had been surprised at how much he needed to take to keep the seizures at bay. He smiled at me. It was that "Kyle with a smile look," and those blue eyes, full of questions, were searching my face.

"Mom, am I going to die?"

"Yes, Kyle. You are dying." My strength came from the Lord. My heart was racing. I had to remain calm. I couldn't cry. I had to be there to help my son. I was breaking apart inside as my heart raced. My own mind was questioning, "Why did it come back? How did it come back? How long does he have?" But I let none of this show.

"Mom, how am I going to heaven?"

I was right next him, on his left side. I held his hand. I sought his face. I was only inches from his beautiful face. I swallowed hard as I forced out a smile. "Kyle, you know how you're going to heaven."

"Mom, I just want to know. How am I going to heaven?"

Puzzled and perplexed on how to answer Kyle, I prayed silently, "Lord, I need you. I need your guidance. I need words for me to say to my son. Give me your strength, Lord. I can't do this!"

I proceeded to ask Kyle, "Kyle, you've accepted Jesus as your Savior, correct?"

"Yes, Mom, you know I have."

"Okay then, Kyle, upon accepting Jesus as your personal Savior and believing that Jesus was born, died, buried and rose on the third day, you have the faith and guarantee of eternal life. You prayed the 'sinners' prayer' and became a child of God's. Do you believe that?"

"Yes, Mom, I do."

I looked at him and still saw a questioning look on his face and in his eyes. "Kyle?"

"Mom, how do I get to heaven?"

I immediately thought of a Scripture verse. I said, "I know what's going on here." I had gotten a tract out of my Bible that went through the plan of salvation. He said he knew all of that and all but didn't know how he was going to get to heaven. I then said that if he believed what I was about to say, he was to repeat after me. He looked at me and quietly nodded in agreement.

"Satan, get behind thee! I walk with the Lord!"

Kyle immediately repeated the phrase. An unbelievable peace filled the room. Calmness came across his face. All questions, all anguish, all fear was gone. In just a moment, after declaring our faith, our belief in the Lord Jesus Christ and quoting scripture to strike down the enemy attack, Kyle was a peace. I was at peace. I reached down and hugged Kyle; he grinned and hugged me so very tightly in return.

There was silence in the room; Kyle quietly spoke to me when I was looking him with a mother's love. "Mom, I still don't know *how* I get to heaven."

I realized in the inflection of his voice on the word *how* what he now meant. How was he going to make his way into the Father's arms? How was he going to go from this life to eternity? But I did not have the answer.

"Kyle, I've never been to heaven. I can't tell you *how* you will get there. But I can tell you *who* will be waiting to hold you, to take your hand, to comfort you, to guide you, to love you, to welcome you—and that is Jesus. Kyle, you get to do something before me. You get to see eternity before I do. You get to see Grammy and Papa before I do. You will be ushered into heaven by loved ones waiting for you to join them."

I wouldn't allow tears to swell in my eyes. I wouldn't allow the sorrow I was feeling to overwhelm me. I wanted Kyle to feel complete, safe, and without fear to creep in and overrun him. Doubt about heaven wasn't an option, and I was doing all I could to help him walk these final days as well as I could.

Kyle was so trusting. He loved the Lord with his whole heart. He was so safe in the comfort of His Father's arms at that moment. I didn't want to believe this was happening. I didn't want my son to die. I wasn't sure how I was going to get through all of this. A part of me was dying as I held my son and assured him that he was going to be okay as he crossed over from earth to heaven.

Kyle quietly said, "Mom, I need to talk to all my brothers and sisters. I want them to know Jesus as their personal Savior. I want them all to accept him as their Lord so they will all be with me in heaven. I know you know the Lord, and you'll make sure Christian does. But, Mom, I need you to talk to my dad."

"Kyle, I don't think I'm the one to do that. I believe you will have to talk to him."

"I don't know what to say to him."

"Kyle, just tell him about your personal relationship with Jesus, how you desire for him to know Jesus as you do. Share what is laid in your heart. God will prompt your dad. You are the seed planter, but Jesus and the Holy Spirit will be the watering and growing agents. Then it is up to your dad to allow them to work in his heart."

So after cuddling and praying, I stepped out to find my other kids who were there for Kyle to talk to them individually about knowing Jesus as their personal Savior. He went beyond his siblings and talked with cousins and others too.

His final days' goal was to bring the glory of the Lord to all who could hear and witness his love for Jesus.

CHAPTER 20

Kyle was having several seizures. They varied in style and length. The staff had decreased his antiseizure medications, believing he was on too high of a dose. They soon learned he wasn't on enough medication and eventually leveled him out.

The one that I experienced with him was a shouting, eyes-closed seizure. Anneliese, Erik, and Dr. Kitchen were present. He just started yelling, "Can I go? Can I go now?"

I wasn't sure what to do or what this exactly meant. I was at his bedside, trying to calm him by touching him, but he just kept on yelling. This was so uncharacteristic of Kyle. I looked at the doctor, and she just sat quietly as though she wasn't sure what to do. He wasn't in any danger or in a position to hurt anyone else. He just kept shouting out things.

I talked to him as I gently touched his arm. Erik had hit the panic button, and some nurses came running in. We all just observed, and I told him, "Yes, you can go."

I didn't know what that meant. It scared me. Was he dying right there? Was this the final moment we'd have with him? But somehow I remained "calm" during this episode. I just assured him that he could go. Eventually he calmed down and slept.

Dr. Kitchen lovingly looked me in the eyes and said I had done a good job with him. She was not the doctor assigned to his care at this time, and he was not in medical distress, so she just let me handle it. She was very proud of how I did. She had not witnessed a seizure of this nature before, either.

After all these seizures, Kyle could no longer keep his head stable, and he required a neck brace to help hold his head upright. He had begun to have double vision, so we patched the worst eye. He joked he was a pirate. His legs were losing their usability quickly. He would want to get up to use the bathroom, but even in just a few hours, he would lose so much use of them it was becoming difficult to help him to the restroom.

The doctors said at first he had months left, but within a day or two, that all changed. The tumors were growing so rapidly, and he was declining so quickly that we figured it was days to weeks. They had cleared him for brain radiation. The dose was for ten days to help reduce the swelling.

This awful, *awful* form of cancer that wasn't known to go to the brain was actually rapidly attacking Kyle's brain and the meningeal lining of his spine. It's as though his body was saying, "I'm home here at Mott. I can relax now. It's time to stop fighting."

So we offered the ten-day brain radiation to Kyle, and he agreed. His body was so thin, frail, and in pain that he needed to be sedated. We walked with him down to the radiation area. He knew these people. After all, he had just undergone twenty days of full-body radiation, just a short half-year or so ago. Kyle joked with them and the staff with him, but the sorrow in their eyes told the sadness they felt seeing him like this.

In order for him to be comfortable, he received as much sedation as they could give without a special team of technicians present. It was to relax him, and basically for the rest of the day, he was so sleepy and groggy that all he did was sleep.

Day 4 arrived. He looked at me and said, "Mom, do you remember when they told me if there ever came a time that I didn't want to do this anymore I could stop?

"Yes, I do."

"I believe that time has come."

I waited for him to say more. I too thought this treatment was too hard on him.

"Mom, it hurts so much to be on that table. I have to get sedation, and it knocks me out for the rest of the day, so I can't enjoy everyone when they are here to see me." He paused. Those beautiful blue eyes had lost their luster. The sorrow, the pain had crept in. He then quietly said, "Mom, we're just delaying the inevitable anyway, aren't we?"

I gently shook my head, as I answered, "Yes, son, we are." Tears were welling up in my eyes.

Then he shared that he'd like today to be his final radiation. He knew they were waiting on him, and Kyle didn't want to let anyone down. "I just want to be able to enjoy everyone. And doing this radiation isn't allowing me to do that," Kyle quietly shared.

"Wow, my son is so strong. He is so full of wisdom and love for others." His health was deteriorating so drastically, and he knew that his life was going to end even with this last radiation. He chose his next course of action. We called for the attending physician to come to his room. Kyle expressed his desire to stop the radiation, and the doctor agreed 100 percent with his decision.

I had a flashback to the time we were sitting in Dr. Jasty's office. She had looked us in the eyes and very deliberately said, "If there ever comes a time that any of us feels the treatment isn't working or it's too hard to endure, we can stop the treatment at any time. This includes parents, doctors, and Kyle."

Kyle remembered those words and made that decision. It was the perfect timing and exactly when he needed to stop all treatments and live his final days happy and awake as much as possible.

CHAPTER 21

How do you say goodbye to your child? Others had come into our lives these final days, people who all loved him but hadn't really been around during the past eighteen months. I understand their want to spend time with him, but I also had to be the one to limit at his request who would be there to see him.

The hospital days were blending into one another. Where did night end and morning begin? I found myself so overtaxed that I literally couldn't function. My brain was shutting down. I couldn't stay awake or operate, and I fell into pure exhaustion in the small family room the staff allowed us to "take over" during this time of crisis.

Kyle's best friend, Peter, and his family came to visit. Kyle tried so hard to stay awake to play cards but kept falling asleep. He would awaken and apologize each time. He had spilled Coke on his t-shirt and was apologetic. Peter and his two brothers just sat patiently, speaking when he'd awaken and joke with him as if nothing was amiss. Kyle knew it was, but this friendship was one of love and admiration. This family, the Curry family, was a gift from the Lord to Kyle, and it extended to Christian as well as me.

Paul, Maddie's dad, came to the hospital and brought a guitar. A Metallica guitar pick was given to Kyle. He tried to strum the guitar, but he was so hot and disoriented, but still polite and appreciative. Maddie was a sweet seven-year-old we came to know on the floor at Mott. Her smile was infectious and her bald head even cuter. She had battled Ewing's sarcoma, and eventually God took her home. Her treatments and Kyle's seemed to correspond almost simultaneously. That's when I got to know her dad, Paul. He and I shared many moments on Mott 7 and the surrounding grounds of the U of M hospital. We shared our battles, tears, and fears.

Kyle's stepmom and I had had some hard moments, but she had been very sweet to Kyle. She always managed to find some of the "coolest" t-shirts for him, like WHO NEEDS HAIR WITH A HEAD LIKE THIS and I'M REALLY EXCITED TO BE HERE and the JOHN 3:16 tie he wore in Anneliese's "fake wedding" the week before her "real" wedding.

I had to get on my knees and ask God for the strength to allow these others to *love on* my boy, when all I wanted was to be the one there for him as it had been for the months previously.

CHAPTER 22

Anneliese was getting married on August 4, 2007, in Lexington, Michigan. We did not feel Kyle was going to be able to attend the wedding, so we had a fake wedding. My sister had gotten in touch with a bridal store, and Anneliese was able to pick out any dress, and they altered it for her to wear. People pulled together and made food, and a cake was provided by the hospital. We held a fake wedding in the chapel one week before the actual ceremony. Kyle was dressed in a suit and tie, and the girls all wore their bridesmaid dresses. The chaplain said he would perform the ceremony, with the exception, of course, of pronouncing them husband and wife.

Kyle was given a pretty daisy bracelet that his stepmom had purchased for him to give to Anneliese. We watched as that replaced the giving of a ring. Kyle was so cute. He beamed with joy and smiled widely. He was wearing a neck brace because his seizures had made the muscles very weak. Once the ceremony was complete, we had a reception on the seventh floor, and everyone came and joined in the celebration! Kyle stated, "This is the marriage before the eyes of God but not recognized by the state of Michigan ceremony." There was no fooling this young man!

*****

The following chapters are excerpts from my journals of our journey.

Hope
August 2007

Hope is a small four-letter word. But a word that holds so much for a family on a cancer journey. I thought of the times I had read scripture: hope for things unseen, hope for the future, hope for the oppressed, hope for the journey, hope, so much to offer.

You take your child to the doctor, hoping that the illness they are experiencing can be quickly and easily treated. A little antibiotic perhaps, and in a few days, all is as good as new. But then you are told it's something more, something that needs more attention. You hope for the best and pray that each test given will provide answers. But then sometimes that test leads to another test, and all the while you are hoping for the best possible outcome. Then there might come a time where the tests reveal something horrific, such as cancer.

We hope the tests are wrong and it can't be as bad as it sounds. We hope the first doctor leads us to the next group of doctors who can lead us to the right diagnosis, which in turn gives us hope that your child will be cured.

We place our hope in the doctors, the tests, and the facility where hopefully the right treatment has been decided. We hope we've made the best educated decision we can. We hope God will answer our earthly prayers and heal the ill child. We hope to leave this terrible illness behind us and move toward the future.

Then, even with all the hope in our hearts, minds and soul, nothing more can be done, our hope changes.

With the help of a chaplain soon after Kyle's relapse in July 2007, I realized what real HOPE is...how it no longer held the same meaning to me. You see, I had lost all hope; it was ripped from my heart, my soul, my very breath. My son was dying; there was no more hope...

The chaplain said, "You still have hope." I gave him a questioning stare as we stood outside those elevator doors. He continued, "Your hope has just changed. It is no longer horizontal, it is now vertical," as he pointed upward.

Peace, tears, joy, all swelled up in my heart upon hearing this great news, HOPE ETERNAL. My hope had not been heavenward. It had been focused on earth. My life was changing in a way I really never truly understood until that moment. Hope eternal, eternal is forever, and this was the way we were looking. Hope in the Lord knowing that He would come and walk my son to join him in his heavenly home. HOPE ETERNAL, what an awesome revelation for me that day.

I've believed on/in the Lord, but heaven seemed like a dream in the fog, not here yet, but look, it was right before my eyes. My son was going to be called to heaven sooner than later, and all eyes were now looking upward, completely waiting for that moment.

*****

Ambulance Ride to Anneliese's Wedding

It seems we associate ambulance rides with bad experiences. Well, I'm here to share with you that not all experiences are sad or bad!

August 4, 2007, was one of the best rides I've experienced, and next to coming back home for the last time, it was Kyle's also! But as I think about it, this ride might have been the cherry on the top of the ambulance rides, after all.

One o'clock! We had watched the clock all morning. Hurry up and get here, 1:00 p.m.

Kyle was dressed in his black I <3 BOOBS t-shirt and his Yankees baseball cap. Earlier he expressed to me, "I'm not wearing a suit, I did that a week ago, and once IS enough!"

The ambulance volunteers arrived promptly, and made sure that all the paperwork was signed and finally Kyle was strapped on the stretcher. The hardest for me at this point were the instructions given to the EMT's. The orders of DNR, "Do not resuscitate," orders that we wished for Kyle. The decision had been made that we would not do anything that prolonged his life when the time came for him to go meet Jesus.

Oh, I need to backtrack a moment and remember the night before! Kyle laid in his hospital bed the night before with a HUGE grin on his face. "I knew I'd get to go!" he quietly said.

Dr. Linda came on duty as his new attending physician that day. I spoke with her in the hallway about my dilemma. I explained that my daughter Anneliese was to be married the next day and I didn't know if I should leave Kyle. He had seemed to stabilize in his health, so that wasn't quite as worrisome. I also knew that he'd put on a good front about all of us being at the wedding, and encourage me to be at the ceremony. Then I expressed to her what he had said to Anneliese when she told him that they would postpone their wedding due to the aggressive deterioration of his health.

"Wouldn't you rather have me there like this than not at all?"

The previous week, when we held the ceremony at the U of M chapel, we didn't know if Kyle would be physically or mentally able to attend the "real" wedding as his health was getting worse by the minute.

I didn't know what to do, and this was one of the most difficult decisions I have ever had to make. Do I leave my son who is dying and attend my daughter's wedding, or do I stay with Kyle and miss her wedding?

Dr. Linda, with eyes wide and questioning, said, "Well, why ISN'T he going?"

"There is no way I can transport him in my van."

She questioned, "Why hasn't an ambulance been ordered? Wasn't his Make-A-Wish gift of minimal value?"

I responded with surprise and explained that no one had suggested it, I didn't think of it, and yes, compared to several others, Kyle's Make-A-Wish didn't require the expense as others had.

Within the hour, she returned with a rather broad smile on her face and said, "They will be here at 1:00 p.m. ready to pick you up!"

Talk about the happiest boy on earth! "I knew I was going to Anneliese's wedding!" He couldn't contain himself! If I didn't know better, I'd believe he was dancing in his bed! His eyes were closed, his smile was ear to ear, and he just let the news sink down into the depths of his soul!

I wasn't allowed to tell anyone that he would be attending the ceremony, except his dad, who was going to come to sit with him at the hospital if I went to the wedding. Gina called me that evening, and she said, "He's coming isn't he?!"

"Well…"

"Oh, Mom, you don't need to say anymore. I can tell he's coming! I can hear it in your voice!"

"Yes, he is, but you can't tell anyone as he wants it to be a surprise!"

Well, the ride from Ann Arbor to Lexington was to take two and a half hours, and that would give me thirty minutes to prepare for the wedding. I should have known nothing would go smoothly for us, and we didn't leave any leeway time in there. Mistake #1, because we had road construction to battle, and lots and lots of traffic!

I chose to sit up front with the driver, hoping that Kyle would try to sleep as we traveled. While sitting up there, I watched the EMT place the GPS on the dashboard. We traveled toward down I-696 and then we had some roadblocks. Recalculate, so we started to go "off roading" and hit some of the parallel streets to keep us moving toward our destination. Turn left here, turn right in 1/2 mile, go in this circle, turn yourself upside down, well, now you know I am exaggerating but that it how it felt as the clock ticked, and I knew we weren't going to make it to the wedding with any time to spare. The driver felt so bad, but we were doing our best to keep moving and not get stuck in traffic. Finally I-94 was in view, and then I saw an I-69 sign, and soon the exit for M-25 toward Lexington signs were in our view! Yes! We were getting closer!

Are we there yet? Through the north end of Port Huron, known as Fort Gratiot, we traveled. Traffic was insane and didn't get any better as we approached Lexington. During the summer, it is a bustling little tourist town, and this weekend in particular was exceptionally busy with their annual art fair lining the main street.

It was nearly 4:00 p.m. when we found the cabins where the wedding was to be held. Guests were being seated as we pulled into the driveway. They were all very surprised at our arrival. I told Kyle I loved him and that I needed to get in and get my dress on and see how Anneliese was doing. I left him in the hands of the EMTs and family, who all came up to greet him.

I later learned his dad and some of the guys kept him company as he waited on his gurney at the altar, where he would witness the wedding and surprise his sister. Kyle was so happy because he had pulled off the surprise, and finally he knew something first before anyone else did!

I did look back at him as I was walking to the cabin, and I saw his million-dollar smile, which was glowing even though he was tired and hurting. He was happy to be at his sister's wedding, the wedding no one thought he would be attending!

God had blessed this day, August 4, 2007, with the most gorgeous summer day one could imagine. There was a warm, a gentle breeze, clear sky, and the water of Lake Huron was the most gorgeous blue and was as smooth as glass. It was as if God was saying, "All's well and I am here. Feel my presence."

Kyle's coordination center was affected, and his body could not regulate very well to different temperatures. God knew, giving us the most perfect day one could have imagined for this very special event. It was a day that would be memorable and comfortable for all.

Trying to remain quiet about Kyle being at the ceremony was not easy to do. Some of the girls had seen the ambulance arrive, but Gina motioned to them that they needed to keep it a surprise.

My daughter looked beautiful. Her sisters had been able to help her prepare for her big day. I kissed Anneliese and told her the traffic was terrible. I didn't mention Kyle but said, "Just give me a minute and I'll throw my dress on and a little bit of makeup too."

Gina came in to help me but really to ask how Kyle was doing. She had kept the secret she learned the night before and was so happy he was here! She whispered, "I could hear it in your voice last night, Mom." I just had that feeling he was going to come! I hugged her and smiled.

The plan was for parasols to help shield the girls as they walked across the yard to the waiting guests. I had to keep pulling the parasol out of Anneliese's dad's hands to try to keep it more in front of her instead of all to the side. I wanted to block the ambulance from her view, as they had parked across the main driveway; and as we were walking out, it was directly in front of us.

Near the approach to the aisle, the umbrella wasn't positioned correctly, and she glanced up, spotting the ambulance! She put her hand to her mouth as she about collapsed to the ground in excitement. I grabbed her arm, and with tears in her eyes, she whispered, "He's here. He's here." I responded with tears and said, "Yes, and he's waiting to see you."

We tried to wipe the tear-stained makeup from under her eyes as our hands shook with excitement and anticipation of the ceremony about to take place. Her father and I walked with her down the aisle, and as pictures revealed, she and I had the same expression on our faces—trying not to cry as we walked happily together to where she would greet her waiting groom.

Lovingly, as she stood to walk toward Tim, Anneliese raise her index finger of her right hand and asked, "Can I have one minute, please?" Tim smiled and nodded his head. She smiled and cried as she went to her brother, who was waiting with a big smile at the end of the groomsmen's line, proudly wearing his BOOBS shirt and Yankees hat and sunglasses of choice! The most precious moment took place at that time. Brother and sister shared a special moment that only a few days earlier we thought would never take place. We are so thankful for the photographs that captured that very precious day not only for my daughter but for our family.

Kyle later shared that he couldn't really see anything from where he was but that he was there and that was the important part! He had made it to his sister's special day, and she would always remember he was there to support her at this wonderful time in her life.

He tried to put on a continuous brave front, but after an hour or so, he needed to be taken to the ambulance so he could rest. It was also air-conditioned, and even though it wasn't hot outside, his body couldn't control his temperature very well. People were kind, but it overwhelmed him too. The IV drugs had begun to wear off, and I had to give him some oral medications. They started to help relieve his pain, and the coolness of the vehicle revived his spirits for a little while more. He questioned why so many people came up to him. I believe he did not understand the magnitude of his appearance on this special day. To him, he was just going to his sister's wedding, like any brother should be doing.

We had several pictures taken, some had tears, some had laughter, but all were marking the day in memory through print. This is the day my entire family came together for the last time before his death.

As mom, I had been so pulled on this wonderful day. The thought of having to choose which child to be with literally had torn my heart apart. I believe it was more so because Kyle had deteriorated so quickly once he was admitted to the hospital. I knew I would have been at least two and on half hours away from him if something would have happened. I learned recently how things can happen all too quickly after the death of my mom.

What if I had arrived in Lexington and received a call he had taken a turn for the worse? What if he went completely blind while I was gone? I knew Fred had said he would be there with Kyle, but I needed to be with Kyle. We had experienced this journey together, every day, every step of the way.

I just cringe and get sick to my stomach every time I think about the decision I thought I was going to have to make, but praise God and a sweet, caring attending physician who did some quick thinking, I didn't have to!

I am so grateful that I mentioned it to Dr. Linda. I had learned to carry so much inside my own heart and head, releasing it all to the Lord over these past few months. The best decision I could think of was to have driven to the wedding, attend the ceremony, and leave immediately following it, but again, I am so thankful that I wasn't required to make that decision.

As I look back at the pictures, tears form in my eyes. There are tears of joy when I see the happiness in my children's eyes at our being together for this beautiful occasion. Then the tears of sadness because I missed out on so much surrounding Anneliese's day, the rehearsal, and in general the preparation for the event. We missed out on staying in the cabins, where we were to enjoy the rustic atmosphere beside one of the beautiful Great Lakes Michigan has to offer.

Then I truly realize what mattered most, what will live on in all our memories, family. Witnessing the union of my daughter and her husband with my children all present, this is what mattered that day.

I remember Kyle saying, "I knew I'd get to go to the wedding. I had faith!"

For the ride home, Kyle requested I sit in the back with him. As I climbed in the back, sitting on the side bench, I looked out the window, watching the wedding festivities continue on. A few friends and families stood near the ambulance saying good-bye. I remember that I couldn't become emotional because this would upset Kyle, and the day had been too grand for that.

We had posed for a family picture, which included my entire family, including my siblings and all of our children. The direct descendants of Robert and Wanda, all together for one last picture. How that tore my heart apart. My last family picture that would include Kyle Robert.

What a difference that makes in how one thinks of life in general. Knowing that one's days are truly numbered, the end was in sight, so to speak, really does change one's perspective.

My heart yearned to continue to celebrate with Anneliese. Life was just beginning for Anneliese and Tim as husband and wife. Yet, here I was going down the driveway with my dying son, knowing his life on earth was coming to a close.

Kyle was in so much pain, and he had managed to stay for four hours after the actual ceremony. He pushed himself to enjoy the wedding that he knew he would be at! And here I was riding in the back of the ambulance with him, feeling very car sick because riding backward and I don't mix! How could I be such a wimp after all he's endured! I sat sideways so I could look forward, and I glanced at Kyle and said, "I must really love you! This is making me very sick!" He looked at my eyes and replied, "Welcome to my world! Now you know how I feel most of the time!" I kissed him and quickly looked out the window. I surely didn't need to throw up all over the place! Only Kyle was allowed to do that!

We were greeted by our Mott 7 family upon our return. Questions and curiosity abounded about our day. They could tell that Kyle was very tired, but he was extremely happy. Oh, he couldn't wait to get his party friends, "Ben and Addy," to help relieve his pain. We had talked with the staff and with each other and turned down the lights, all ready to settle in after our very long and exciting day.

I was just falling asleep when I heard, "Mom, Mom, come here!"

I jumped up and went to Kyle's bed side. I said, "What? What's wrong?" He had sounded so urgent it had alarmed me.

"Mom, Mom, come here," were the words he said as he motioned for me to get closer so he could talk right to me, look into my face.

Our faces were inches apart from each other, and he said, "Mom, everyone says I'm such a good boy. But, Mom, I couldn't be such a good boy if I didn't have such a good mom. Mom, do you hear me?"

With tears streaming down my face, I said, "Yes, honey, I hear you. Thank you."

Grabbing me tighter, he said, "Mom, this is ME talking, not the drugs. Do you hear me? It's me, Mom, not the drugs. Remember this, Mom, remember it always. I love you."

I hugged him, thanked him, and told him how much I loved him. We smiled, and I said, "It's time to sleep now."

"Okay," he said and closed his eyes.

About ten to fifteen minutes later, as I was dozing off, I heard, "Mom, Mom!"

I jumped up and asked, "What is it Kyle?" and quickly moved to his side.

"Remember what I said a little bit ago?"

"Yes," I said as I touched his face.

He then said, "Mom, come close, please." So as I stared in his beautiful blue eyes again, he focused very intently. (You see, he could only see with one eye, and that was very minimal.) "Mom, it's me, not the drugs. Remember that, please remember what I said." I hugged him tightly and reassured him and then got him resettled in his bed.

The next day, after our family returned from the wedding, Kyle looked at me and asked me as quietly as can be, "Mom, do you remember what I told you last night?"

"Yes, I do."

"Mom, it was me talking not the drugs. Always, remember that." His gaze was so deep into my eyes. It was as though he were afraid that I hadn't believe it was truly him talking. It was his way of paying me the highest compliment I could ever receive in my lifetime.

Kyle knew how my life had gone. How so many hadn't appreciated me but he did. He made sure I knew it was him, that it came from the depth of his heart and soul.

He told me not to ever feel guilty because he had had cancer. He was so kind and loving. "Mom, we did everything they asked," he would say. I'll tell you I tried really hard not to let guilt take over, and to this very day, it still sneaks into my inner being and has tried to destroy me. Why didn't I get him to the doctor earlier? Why didn't I notice the tumor in his abdomen? Why, why, why? Not why did this happen, or why didn't I notice anything?

I did ask Dr. Jasty about one week after his relapse a question, "If I had gotten Kyle to the doctor sooner, do you think it would have made a difference?" She lovingly reassured me that had I taken him in earlier, they probably wouldn't have felt anything. You see, the Lord had laid on my heart back in November of 2005 to "prepare for cancer and diabetes." Why didn't I take him in then? That's where my guilt eventually took me. And it still can on really bad days.

Two weeks earlier than Kyle's original doctor's appointment he had come home from his dad's house and playing football and he was complaining about pain in his side. I think if only I had gotten him in then...

I shared my thoughts with the doctor, and she lovingly said to me that even then, the cancer was probably quite progressed. It was just so hard to hear what she said next. With tears in her eyes and a look that was so sad, she said that the medical community thought Kyle was going to be the first one to survive DSRCT after having it on his liver. I looked at her quizzically and listened to her next words. You see they've never had anyone who had it on their liver survive for any length of time.

Do you know how the feeling is when your throat falls to the pit of your stomach as though the floor opened up and swallowed you whole? That's what happened at that moment to me. "What?" I managed to say. She just looked at me as we sat there holding hands.

I remember at that moment how so very happy I was that she hadn't told us that statement earlier. Kyle fought, Kyle laughed, and Kyle lived to the fullest he could. Had we been told up front that his chances were even less for survival, I'm not sure how the previous months would have played out.

My mind went to an event that happened earlier in his treatment. One mother, Michele Hill, had approached me and asked me to please talk to her. We went into a small lounge. She asked me if I had Kyle's funeral all planned out. I was a little taken back by the comment, as it had not ever entered my mind. I responded, "No, I do not think of that." I am a realist, and I knew it was a very strong possibility, but no, I had not thought of planning a funeral for my son. She confided in me that she had her daughter's all planned.

How the irony of life goes. Approximately a year later, my son was dying and her daughter was in full remission, headed off to college.

"Mom, don't feel guilty."

CHAPTER 23

It seems we associate ambulance rides with bad experiences. Well, I'm here to share with you that not all experiences are sad or bad!

I had to make a decision. The wedding was done. The hospice team was brought in. Kyle could no longer walk; the vision loss had subsided. It was time to go home. As we road in the ambulance to our little two-bedroom duplex we called home, Kyle slept much of the way. I, on the other hand, needed to look out the window so I didn't get car sick. This is our last ambulance ride together; no, this is our final vehicle ride of any type together.

Heather had sent balloons to the house for Kyle's greeting home. They were waiting for us upon our arrival, along with Anneliese, Gina, and other family members.

The hospital bed was placed in the living room. A WELCOME HOME, KYLE banner was hanging on the wall beside the bed. Hospice personnel arrived with the supplies we'd need to use for this duration. Kyle had seemingly taken a turn for the better, to everyone's surprise. Apparently, the four days of brain radiation had done some good at stopping the tumors' growth at a rampant rate for now. We were given more days than the doctors had hoped. They thought he only had a few days, but you know, we never know what God will do.

The instructions were given, the training of administering the medication we could give was done, and we were home. The house seemed to be a revolving door. This one coming, that one going, Kyle craving one of his fast-food items to munch on, causing someone to quickly run out and grab it for him. Usually, only a bite or two was taken, but it made him so happy.

Don, a former husband of mine, came to visit often and had a group from Homer Methodist Church come and sing songs for Kyle. Usually they just gather outside, especially on a warm summer day, but the rain wanted to drip, so all these people made it into our tiny home and sang wonderful, comforting songs to Kyle and all of us actually. "Lord I Lift Your Name on High" was a special song of Kyle's, and he even sang along with them. He was lying there with his eyes closed much of the time, as his vision was that of a periscope out of one eye only. He just cherished the moments. I could tell he was becoming sleepy, but he never complained or asked them to leave.

One of his favorite nurses drove from Toledo to visit him at our home. He was having awful hallucinations at this time and felt so poorly about it. He would look at Marnie and say something like, "I'm sorry. I know they're not real." He'd tell us this even in the midst of the episode. Marnie said she hadn't known anyone to be aware and alert during an episode while they were having a hallucination and then try to stay as clear as possible in their thought process. That's just Kyle—a mystery and a trooper!

The hallucinations were increasing in number and length. I was with him around the clock. This particular one lasted several hours. He'd talk about the blood and bicycle handles through his legs and then comment, "I know they're not there, but I can't help what I see." We didn't know how to help him. I would sit by his bed and hold his hand, administer medications, and reassure him he was okay and that we were there with him. That someone would be with him at all times. He would never be left alone.

The hospice nurse came out and raised his dose of pain medications, and he finally fell asleep, so I went directly to the bedroom and slept for the next three hours. We were both exhausted as this episode was over four hours. His dad was actually there to witness what I'd been going through over the past few days and weeks. For some reason, when his dad would visit in the evening, Kyle could pull it all together. He'd laugh and joke and listen to conversations and join in. He was always up and alert during these evening hours from six to nine. It's like his brain took over and said it was going to be the best it could be during these times because he wanted to enjoy family time.

I had to be the buffer, and Kyle finally told me the people he wanted to have stop in and visit him and those he chose not to have visit. He specifically asked for certain ones to stay away because he said that they just looked at him like a piece of furniture. He expressed how he was still himself, but it was as though they were looking through him, not at him as a person. This was extremely hard for me to do, as it appeared I was picking and choosing, but in actuality, I was honoring the wishes of my dying son.

Kyle loved to have Christian up by him on the bed. However, as the pain became worse, Christian could only stand by him and lean on the railing. They would hold hands, or Kyle would reach out to touch Christian's face. One of the many conversations that took place that was so very precious was when Kyle talked to Christian about dying. He told him that if he ever wanted him to see what he was doing after he died, Christian only have to say his name and ask for him to come and look. Kyle told him he'd be able to see what Christian was doing. Christian wanted to know if he could see what Kyle would be doing, and Kyle told him, "No, buddy you won't be able to." Kyle was so sensitive to his little brother and said, "How do I tell him about dying?"

A precious conversation between the boys was when Kyle talked to Christian about Jesus. He affirmed that Christian knew Jesus and that "Mom will make sure you know Jesus personally, and one day you'll be with me in heaven. She'll make sure you know all about him."

Anneliese and Gina, along with my nephew, learned to "push meds" to give me a break. Heather and Darren didn't come visit as often or stay. It was so hard for them to see their brother so sick. If Kyle called them or expressed he wanted them to come, they did. Heather and Brad had done just that when he was at Mott. They drove late into the night because he just needed to see them.

It's like he desperately just needed to see Christian. His vision was failing. He was losing the sight in his second eye. He took my hand and asked for me to please get Christian there to the hospital. He wanted to see him. I told him he just left yesterday, that he *had* seen him. Kyle knew he had, but insisted that he needed him brought back to the hospital that day to see his brother. Christine and I met halfway between Midland and Ann Arbor on the expressway.

I brought Christian into the room, and Kyle had him get on the bed and just stared at him, touching his face, caressing him. Kyle was afraid he was going to be blind within a very short time and wouldn't ever "see" his brother again. God was so good. Kyle's vision loss was apparent in one eye, but the other eye maintained a small circle of vision. He also was experiencing some hearing loss, but it was restored.

The hallucinations caused so much pain to his body.

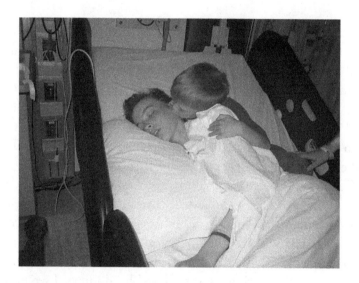

CHAPTER 24

The final week

I had cemetery lots given to me back in 1989. They are at Memorial Gardens on Meridian Road, or as we say M-30. My parents are buried there. My grandparents are buried there. The older cemetery is Homer Cemetery, where the bulk of my mother's family ancestors reside. Fred looked into that cemetery, but then agreed for Kyle to be buried in one of the plots I have at Memorial. It didn't cost us extra. It is so sad to even think about this having to bury my son. That is not the order of life. Parents are to die first, not children.

The two lots were given to me by a family friend, Mabel, as she had moved out of the area. I actually had gotten them a few months before my eldest daughter, Heather, was hit by a car in December 1989. I thought she was going to need to use one of them at that time. Her accident, which involved her being hit by a car in front of my home and suffering a severe closed-head injury, I see now was God's way of preparing me for this time with Kyle.

There were so many moments Kyle was going through that I understand from Heather's injury. The brain is a remarkable organ. As the tumors were growing in number and size, I saw much of what I had prepared for with Heather. Although not the same, Kyle's tumors were taking over his brain, and his responses were very similar to Heather's head injury. Heather was hit by a car in 1989, and she sustained a severe head trauma, along with various broken bones. She is a walking miracle. Her various stages of coming out of the coma gave me the insight I needed to see in Kyle as he was slowly going into a coma-like state. It was reverse, but I believe God used Heather's accident as a guide for me during Kyle's dying process.

The day came, and Fred and I had to go to the funeral home. Gina and Anneliese stayed with Kyle. I told him I had some errands to run. I didn't lie. I didn't plan on lying. I just couldn't tell him where I was going. We had decided it would be the two of us going into the funeral home. We needed to make decisions. However, it was easy, in the sense that Kyle had already shared with me what he wanted. "Mom, I want a blue casket, like Grammy had." So a blue casket is what we ordered.

The funeral home was in a home atmosphere. The city of Midland was busy doing road construction, and it was a mess to get into the funeral-home parking lot. So it was decided that we would hold the visitation and funeral at the Baptist Church we attended. It was large enough and could hold the visitors we expected.

Fred had me pick out the saying on the little memorial cards we would have for people to take to remember Kyle. He said, "You've always been better at that stuff." It didn't take long for the right one to touch my heart.

All in all, the appointment was very quick. It helped, and hurt my heart, that I had just been there four months earlier to make the final arrangements for my mother. Also, knowing Dave, the funeral homeowner and director, made it all flow as easily as possible. He asked some very hard questions. Did I want the wisps of hair Kyle had left shaved off? Did I have any special requests? I found myself praying as I sat in my car to go in and talk to him. And within a few minutes, all the arrangements were made, and I was walking out, with plans to meet later to go over flowers. I was crying...tears slowly leaking from my eyes. My son was dying; I just made plans for his final burial—for him to be laid to rest after his soul goes to be with the Lord.

I walked into the flower store Fred and I had agreed to. My heart stopped. His wife was there and picking out flowers. I did not react very well.

"No! This is *my* son, Fred, and my son...not hers." I didn't want my son's final plans to be made by another woman. Inside I was screaming, "She's not his mom! I am!"

I got after Fred and asked why she was here, as we had agreed this was our responsibility for Kyle, just the two of us! He tried to calm me down and felt she knew more about flowers than he did.

I understand. She is his stepmom and has treated him well, but *he* is *my son*, not *hers*! I gave birth to him. I watched him grow. I watched him flourish. I watched him get sick. I watched him cry, puke, have diarrhea and she didn't even have a clue about all the requests he had made concerning his final days. I had to try to honor his requests, so why did I have to allow her to help with his final flowers?

The flowers were ordered, paid for, and just waiting for that call—that call that my son had died. Oh Lord, how can this be? How can Kyle be really dying? I was doing all the motions, but my heart ached so terribly!!

Upon arriving back at the house, Kyle was napping. When he awoke, he asked where I had been. I looked out the window, the sun was shining, the living room door opened; it was a warm late summer day for all of us to enjoy.

I looked into Kyle's beautiful blue eyes, and they were searching mine. "Mom, where did you go?"

A deep breath, a big sigh, a loving look, and a quick prayer, "Oh, God, please give me the words needed to tell my son where I've been." I began to say, "You know, Kyle, I've never lied to you during this whole process, and I'm not about to now." I took his hand in mine as I prepared to tell him exactly where I had been. I proceeded to share how we had picked out his casket, the memorial card, and that his funeral and viewing would be at Midland Baptist, etc.

He looked at me and said, "It sounds nice. It's like Grammy's casket, right?"

I assured him it was as close as we could get. I smiled, through tears and a heart that was breaking on the inside, to assure him I did the best I could.

"Mom, at the cemetery, I want the lot that is closest to Grammy and Papa! I think I should get the first pick since I'm dying first. I want to be near them." He grinned.

That little stinker! He knew how to break up a hard subject with just a few words. I laughed, hugged him, and agreed he could be in the lot closest to my parents.

Then out of nowhere came "So, Mom, what am I wearing when I die?"

"That's a good question! Do you have any ideas?"

"Mom, I'm wearing a t-shirt, not a suit! Suits are just not me. Is that okay?"

"Kyle, you may wear whatever you'd like. I'd never put you in a suit. That's just not you."

"But, Mom, everyone I see always has on a suit. Won't people get mad or upset?"

"No, son, they won't. So now, what t-shirt do you prefer to wear? And what pants, regular or pajama pants?"

"I will wear my black stretchy pants, you know, the kind I like."

So I went and pulled out the pair of pants he was talking about. I also grabbed a handful of t-shirts as he had numerous to choose from.

"Mom, I want the one that has the poker stuff on it—no, how about the one that says something about a bald head as good-looking as this, who needs hair?"

Laughing, I agreed with him. He surely was good looking with or without hair. Then I found the shirt I thought he might like. The shirt said, I'M REALLY EXCITED TO BE HERE.

"What do you think?" I asked him as I held it up for him to see as he lay in his bed.

"Perfect!" was his response! That "Kyle with a Smile" grin was from ear to ear!

"People will laugh when they come up to the casket! I want them to laugh...you see, 'Hahaha, I'm really excited to be here, lying in a casket...not! *But* I am really excited to be in heaven with Jesus! And that is where I'll be when people walk up to the casket!"

I laughed with him, and his contagious sense of humor just warmed my soul! So the matter was settled, and those clothes were set apart, not to be worn again until his final viewing and burial.

CHAPTER 25

I have to admit I had a very hard time picking out the flowers for the funeral. Fred and I were to be there, but he had brought his wife. I was not handling it well. One of my girls came and planned on just listening and being supportive, and if Fred's wife had done the same, I would have been okay. However, she started picking and having an opinion. I was very upset, and my sadness and patience was let loose. I am not proud of my reaction, but this was *my* son, our son, not hers. I was buying my son's funeral flowers—flowers to put on his casket, flowers to say my final earthly farewell. I finally settled down, and we were able to figure things out. The tears were so real, so deep. The lump in my throat, the held-back emotions, the panic, the reality that my son was dying—it all came to a realization. My Kyle Robert was not going to be on this earth much longer.

Kyle had asked that we not make his casket look trashy but had requested a few things to be placed with him. A John Deere Green item, M&M's (like his papa had), you know, just some special memorabilia.

The kids were usually there in the evenings. They would watch the television show *The Office*, and Anneliese would remind Kyle of the scene. He couldn't see the TV but had his eyes closed and would say such and such was going to happen and laugh out loud, and he was right.

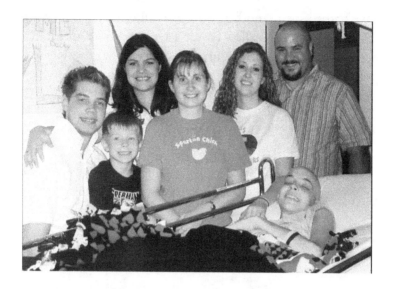

The pain became so real and frequent. His hallucinations became so real, lengthy, and unbearable for him. He would want me and only me. I would stand with him, watching him move ever so slightly because it hurt so horribly. We were watching for possible seizures; with the growing tumors, he was in such pain.

In a moment of playfulness, Kyle would joke with everyone around him. How he managed to pull himself together when his dad came around amazed me, like there was nothing wrong, nothing hurts, etc. But as soon as he was gone, Kyle would ask for medications and want to sleep.

I find myself so tired. Although the kids were there to help, Kyle still wanted Mom.

The day came when Kyle said, "Mom, I need to sleep my way to meet Jesus."

I called the hospice nurse with his request. You see, he was too tired, too sore, tired of the hallucinations that he knew were hallucinations but had no control over. It was just time to sleep.

My heart was hurting, and my mind was screaming, "No, no, no! Not yet, please! But knowing he was in so much pain—pain I couldn't take for him or away from him—I knew this was the right move.

We had all spent another few private moments with Kyle while he was still aware and called Pastor Payne to come and join us in prayer. He and his wife, Tracy, arrived after Kyle was heavily sedated. We prayed, cried, and loved on him and each other.

The house was quiet after a little while—too quiet.

CHAPTER 26

The television was on. The kids were watching *The Office*, but the quietness was eerie. We took turns holding his hand, sitting by him, but he just lay there in his bed. I promised him that he would *never* be alone.

I was beginning to mourn silently. "My son is gone. My son is no longer with me." My heart was beating to a sadness I could not put into words, and my tears were starting to well up. My mind kept saying, "It's over."

This is the day the world stopped for me. This is what the future looked like. This is not supposed to be happening. My child is not supposed to die. My child is only fifteen and a half years old; he was supposed to be looking forward to driver's training, to high school, college, a career—not into the face of Jesus in heaven!

As we all sat, it was so noticeable—the silence. No more "Kyle with a Smile," no more laughter or corny jokes, no more "Please run to Taco Bell" or "Can I have…" You name it, a special food, but no more.

Kyle's heart was still beating, but his life was gone. We administered his meds, teasing him about Benny and Addy and Morphy. I placed my hand on his bald head. It did have a few slight wisps of hair. I could feel his pulse at the top of his head, you know like where the baby's soft spot is located. It just pulsated in a slow rhythm. Those horrific tumors were swelling inside this beautiful boy's head, causing the whole bed to move with the pressure inside of his slight body that barely worked.

I began to pray with all my heart. "O God, thank you for the last six to eight weeks we were given! Thank you, Lord, for the time we had with Kyle and the goodness and kindness of his heart and personality. God, I know he was your child before he was mine." I kept repeating claims I know were good. "God you are in control. You have a *plan*!" I didn't like God's plan, but I prayed over and over in my mind for Him to give Kyle comfort, to give us comfort, to *hold* us so tight we would remain strong in Him!

Gina, Anneliese, and I took turns sleeping on the couch. Kyle's breathing was steady, quiet throughout the night and day. We talked to Kyle, even though he was unresponsive. When my dad died, I learned that the hearing is the final sense to go. I talked about Christian and his school day; actually, I talked to him as though he were able to respond.

Twenty-four hours had passed. The house was just too still. Fred came by; the girls were in and out. We noticed his breathing pattern changing about midnight. I phoned Fred and suggested he come back. It didn't look good.

He and Penny came by. Fred sat facing Kyle as he was lying more on his right side. I was behind Kyle just touching his arms or head—just touching him very gently—when out of nowhere, Kyle's eyes opened. Yes, they *opened*!

"Do you know Jesus Christ as your Savior?" he said very clearly, looking directly into his father's face.

Shock and disbelief came over my body. I sat wide eyed and gently looked at Kyle's face. He was intently staring into his dad's face. Fred looked at me.

"He's asking you. He knows I know the Lord," I prompted.

Fred answered his son's question. "Yes, I accepted the Lord…"

Kyle closed his eyes. His body relaxed. He was unconscious again.

I gently touched and loved on my son. His breathing became regular. We sat. We waited. He had normal breathing respirations, no longer labored or shallow. Fred decided to go home, as it looked like we were going to "get through another night."

I sat in the dimly lit room. Fred was the person I was to get to Kyle, the person he was waiting to talk to about Jesus. He was the reason "he couldn't get through the gates on Friday when he thought he was dying." All this time, now early hours on Tuesday, Kyle was waiting to hear that his father had received Christ as his Savior. He knew now that his dad would one day be in heaven too.

Monday found us all just sitting and waiting. Christian was off to school; I was trying to have him lead a normal life. He didn't need to be around all day waiting. I felt he needed to try to have some type of normalcy during this very long period of waiting.

I was giving IV meds to Kyle about 2:30 a.m. to 3:00 a.m. on Tuesday, September 18. The stream of light from my bedroom was enough to light the area I needed to see. The girls were sleeping on the couch and loveseat, and I was so very quiet they didn't know I was administering his medications.

I was slowly pushing the medication and thinking, "Not too fast, buddy. I'm being careful, and I don't want to make your tummy sick." You see, the nurses at U of M talked about how the meds would leave a taste in children's mouths, and they would sometimes throw up. Kyle told me about the taste previously, so I was so very careful.

Kissing sounds? I shook my head. Kissing sounds again! As I looked down at Kyle, I saw a faint smile and opened eyes. How could this be? He was so severely sedated, yet here he was looking at me with a beautiful, faint smile.

"Hi buddy!"

He just gazed at me. He tried to smile a little more, but then just made kissing sounds again.

"Do you want a kiss?"

He slowly, very slowly, and gingerly moved his head in a very slight nodding motion.

I bent down and kissed his cheek. He looked at me with seeking eyes, yearning for me to do more. He was trying to tell me something. His head briefly moved with a side to side motion, as if saying "No!"

I realized he wanted to kiss me, and I said with a tear, "Oh, you want to kiss me!"

Kyle, with the smile, did just that, and I bent down, and we kissed. I had been so aware of germs I was afraid to kiss him on the lips, but he wanted to give his mama a kiss—a real kiss. Tears leaked from my eyes. The joy I felt was priceless, unexplainable. I told him how much I loved him and was so proud of him. He made another very quiet kissing sound.

I asked if he wanted to kiss his sisters. He smacked again, and I woke his sisters so he could kiss them too. He quickly fell back asleep. We awoke in the morning to give more meds and get Christian off to school.

CHAPTER 27

The morning routine was off to a good start. Gina, Anneliese, and I were getting things around for the day when the hospice nurse and an aide arrived at the house at about 9:30 a.m. They were going to bathe Kyle and turn him. I was very nervous about moving him, especially since I knew the swelling in his neck and brain from the tumors were so much worse. When you can feel the pulse of your child through the top of his head, it can't be good.

They began to prepare Kyle for his sponge bath, and as they turned him, he began shaking violently. The nurse yelled for someone to grab the syringe of meds in the fridge. There was a lot of commotion, but with everyone's quick reactions, within a matter of just a minute or so, the seizure was under control. My heart was racing, and tears were streaming down my face. The girls were scared yet reacted in a timely manner, knowing we had syringes of meds ready for just this reason. We had hoped never to use them, but so thankful they were there and ready to be used if necessary. Standing back, I watched the situation. I couldn't move; I just watched his body violently shaking, so lifeless yet rigid. "O God, please calm this seizure," I prayed.

Kyle was lifeless. The medication given to him stopped the seizure. They laid his body back down. We all stopped and took a breath. The hospice nurse was definitely shaken up; this is exactly what we were trying to avoid, a seizure to this magnitude. Phone calls were made to the physician, and more sedative medications were administered. My heart was beating out of my chest; the knowledge that there was absolutely nothing I could do to help my son was tearing me apart inside. I stood by helplessly, or at least that's how I felt. I didn't feel like I got to the fridge in time to do any good, but we did. The seizure stopped. Kyle was safe, as were the nurse and the aide.

The day slowly ticked on. The silence in the room was deafening. We all knew that his last breath was nearer now than it had ever been. People came and went, quietly whispering into his ear their final words they wanted to express to him. I was so very grateful that we had had time to tell him things that we wanted him to hear—to tell him how much we loved him, to tell him how very proud we were of him, and to tell him he would forever live among us. Some don't get to tell their loved ones precious thoughts or words they wish to say as the person is dying. We were blessed that he had been awake and mentally aware enough to understand and cherish those moments just a few days previously. These final words were for us, and we were praying he heard them too. Hearing is the final sense to go. I believed deep down Kyle Robert was listening, hearing every word we spoke. Scripture was read, songs were sung, and love was surrounding him.

Kyle's dad was there until late into the evening. He went home, and Anneliese went home. She wasn't able to sit and watch her baby brother any longer. It was too hard to be waiting—just waiting for that moment, that moment of his last breath.

CHAPTER 28

Gina and I sat in the living room. Christian was tucked away in his room for the night. As I thought about Christian, I thought about how he was going to handle everything. He was there day and night. He sat with the big kids; he sat with Kyle and lay by him as he was able.

Christian played the Game Boy that Kyle had given him when he received the PSP from his eighth-grade class. Christian's eyes were showing signs of stress. His right eye was turning inward. I saw it happening over the past six to eight weeks. I had too much on my plate to have him checked out, and it seemed to be better in the morning.

Kyle had spoken with Christian about his dying. I reflected on those words he had said—the words of a dying brother trying to take care of his precious little brother.

"Am I going to be able to see you?" Christian asked.

"No, but I will be able to see you. All you have to do is say my name, and I'll come down and watch what you're doing."

"He's a remarkable young man," was all I kept thinking. "He is the one dying, and all he cares about is us, his family." He wanted to make sure we were all going to be okay. He told me not to cry at his funeral. That I couldn't guarantee him but said I'd sure try. We weren't to wear black, and all his cousins on my side of the family, along with his siblings, were to wear Beatles t-shirts at his funeral. He had it all planned out. He spoke with each one about the Lord and his salvation for each one because he wanted to make sure that we would all get to heaven one day with him.

"Mom, I'm not scared to die." Even in the private moment, when I kicked everyone out for some "Mom and me" time just a few days ago, he shared with me once again, "No, Mom, I'm not scared." He did share during this precious time about some things that he had spent time on that he felt weren't good. They were not God-honoring. He shared that playing Pokemon was not good. He went into a very private conversation with me at that time. He then said he needed to go before the Lord with his concerns He went before the Lord in prayer and, when he was done, instructed me to throw away every item associated with Pokemon—everything, right then and there, that very moment. I did as I was instructed. He explained how it was evil and asked I was to never ever allow Christian to play it. Kyle had almost everything affiliated with Pokemon; this included things that probably had some monetary value to them also. He was just very strong in his instructions about disposing everything. Once he was assured they were in the trash, a peace came over him, and he smiled.

"Mom, don't spoil Christian. Don't give him everything he wants or asks for. It won't be good for him if you do." He was the big brother, but he was the daddy image for Christian too. He had cried, "Mom, I won't be here to help him. I won't be here to grow up with him." The tears flowed and flowed because he was failing his little brother by not being there for him.

I had assured him that it is the first five years of a child's life that set the tone and affect him the most. He was in Christian's life; he was the main "man" in his life and had helped shape, direct, and raise him with me. I assured Kyle that Christian would always have him in his heart and mind. The fact that Kyle had shown Christian how much he loved the Lord was the biggest lesson he could ever teach him. It was the best legacy he could ever leave him with. Christian was given the best five years any little boy could ask for having a big brother like Kyle. He was kind, compassionate, giving, loving, humorous, gentle, loving, and so much more. Kyle had given in so many ways to his little brother, and Kyle felt at peace when we finished talking.

My son, Kyle Robert, had made sure all of us were taken care of. He had thanked me for being a good mom, telling me he couldn't be a good boy if I hadn't been a good mom. He told me the glimpse of heaven he had seen; he was walking us to heaven with him. He excused his brother Darren and sister Heather for not being with him as much as the other two older siblings.

"Mom, don't be hard on Darren and Heather. If it were reversed, I don't know how much I could be with them either. It's okay, Mom. I know they love me."

The thoughts and memories of the last few days and weeks just flooded my mind as I sat there. My baby's head was pulsating so hard; those awful tumors were raging in his whole body. I remembered his conversation with his siblings about his bodily functions. We were giving him stool softeners, and he had said something like he'd make a mess anyway after he dies. How many fifteen-year-old dying boys would joke about something like this? Only my Kyle. He always brought humor into our everyday life and knew just how to lighten the mood.

CHAPTER 29

Gina and I decided we would take turns staying awake through the night of the eighteenth of September. About midnight, we started to hear raspy sounds, that gargled breathing we knew well from being with my parents in their final hours. Mom had just passed away in April, so death was fresh to our family. Gina had been by her side, and the boys and I had walked in on her last breath. Kyle had looked at me and said something like, "Mom I want my eyes closed as well as my mouth when I die." I had to swallow hard when he told me this. I had no control over any of that but assured him I would see that I would do my best.

I would find myself in the bedroom or the basement in tears. My tears were usually filled with silent crying as best I could so no one knew or heard the sorrow I was feeling. It was so hard to keep going, to keep keeping on, to keep placing one foot in front of the other, but God gave me strength. God gave me comfort; I could feel his arms encircle me. I had to answer questions that I never thought I'd hear, questions and comments no mother should ever have to endure. But I felt blessed to be able to have those times too. Other mothers never get those last moments, days, or weeks with their children. I was blessed. In the midst of this heart turmoil, unfathomable circumstance, I was blessed.

I remembered so many little details from the past few weeks. The tenderness Kyle had with Christian even when he was hurting so much just warmed my heart. I pray that Christian remembers the softness his brother held for him, the love he held for him. The memory of Kyle may slip away slowly, but I *must* keep it alive for

Christian! Not to live in a grief-stricken manner but to *live*! To know that his brother loved the Lord so very much and that he loved him too. To know that his brother cared more about him and was in tears that he wouldn't be there to help raise him to become a man of God. My fifteen-year-old son is/was a man of wisdom, love, patience way above his age. I need to remember these moments for Christian, so he would always know that Kyle loved him more than life itself!

*****

I captured my thoughts and listened to the room sounds as we sat in silence. The only noise was the breathing sounds Kyle was making. He was making gurgling noises. We could hear the slow and shallow breathing, as we sat and watched his chest rise and fall. Gina sat on one side of his bed, while I sat on the other. I wanted so to climb in bed with him, hold him, and tell him he was going to be okay. I couldn't. I was afraid to move him since his seizure in the morning. I didn't want to do anything that might set him into another shaking, jarring motion. He lay there, we held his hand, we stroked his face, we whispered to him.

"It's okay. It's okay to go be with Jesus." These were hardest words I could ever speak, the words I really didn't want to say but knew I must. I needed to let my baby know that when Jesus came to walk him to heaven, I was right there with him. I was saying and doing all I could to help release him from this fallen world's grip, this world that is full of evil, pain, suffering, and sorrow that had allowed his body to be overrun with cancer. However; the evil had never won his spirit or love for the Lord. The truth is, God had won! So many had followed our journey, many had come to know Christ, many had reached out in humanity to Kyle and our family with a love most never get to see or experience. We had a glimpse of heaven just four days ago when Kyle went into another dimension and shared with us what he saw, who he saw, and how beautiful heaven was at its gates.

Kyle was sure today was going to be the day—the day he finally was going to be with Jesus! He had me call everyone to get them there. He was pretty sure Anneliese was not going to make it from

SVSU once we got her out of her class, but he asked for us to try and to tell her to hurry.

His eyes would glass or glaze over, and he would seem to be *somewhere else* at times. Anneliese was released from class, as her professors all knew her brother was in the final stages of life. She hurried and made it home in record time.

"Mom, the grass is a green I have never seen before!" he exclaimed. He motioned for me to get closer to him and in a whisper, he said, "Mom, it's so green!"

He was looking off as if in a different world. Slowly, he said, "Grandma Miller?" and a puzzled expression formed on his face. Then a smile broke out, and he laughingly said, "Hi Grammy! I didn't know you could ride a bike! Okay, I'll see you soon!"

Kyle's eyes became unglazed, and as he refocused to the room, he looked at me and asked, "Who is Grandma Miller? She said she'll see me soon!"

I had chills come over my body. I looked at him and explained that Grandma Miller was his papa's grandma, a grandma he had never heard about or would even remember if he had, as he was only eight when my dad died.

He began to tell us about seeing Grammy riding a four-person bike and was laughing and smiling. She too had said she would see him soon. Kyle went on to explain about the view he saw, the view of the greenest grass he had ever seen, and then described it as a color so unlike any we know here on earth.

He asked me to come close to him, so I bent down once again and got right close to his face. "Mom, I got to the gates, and they won't let me in. Mom, I can't wait to go. Who am I supposed to talk to about Jesus? Get them here soon so I can go!"

I responded I didn't know, but God would lead us to the person he's supposed to talk to, I was sure of that. I was thinking, "Son, I have no idea who you are supposed to still reach."

"Mom, there was a big hotel, a hotel bigger than I have ever seen. The rooms are all bright and shiny. Mom, get whoever I am supposed to talk to here. I want to go!"

I assured Kyle that I would do my best to figure out who he was still supposed to talk to about Jesus. He felt reassured and rested peacefully. In the meantime, we had all gathered, except for his dad, whom we had not been able to reach via either of his phones. That was very frustrating to Kyle. He wondered why people had cell phones if they weren't going to answer them and shared how he had never wanted one. His dad had gone to work in Lansing and either had not heard his phone or had it turned off. Kyle talked to him later that evening, teasingly yet seriously, about "what's the use of having a cell phone if you are not going to answer it?"

I looked at Gina. "Do we call Fred?" He had just left an hour or so ago. We were told each person dies a little differently. The very young, the middle aged, and the old aged die or sustain differently. I had experienced my parents' moment of death; I was there for their last days, hours, and breaths. I didn't know if this was the end for Kyle. I didn't know how long we had.

The gurgles in his throat, the death sound was there, but his heartbeat was regular. We sat. I was being selfish; I was okay with it just being Gina and me there and Christian in his room if this was the time for Kyle to pass from earth to heaven. I was holding my boy's hand. I didn't want to let go to use the phone. I promised him I would be there, and that is a promise I was going to keep.

We sat, silently prayed, and just gazed upon that sweet boy's face. The sounds lessened; the breathing became clear again. We looked at each other. This was not the moment Kyle was going to die.

As I continued to sit near him, Gina went to the loveseat. We decided to take turns staying awake. She was going to see if she could get a little sleep. As she lay there, I slowly moved to the couch just a couple feet away. I was still close to him, but more comfortable than the stools we sat on by his bed.

Gina said, "Mom, do you see that?"

"What?"

"The bright light moving around outside," she responded.

"No, but do you feel the presence of angels. Or of spiritual beings, the Lord?"

I could feel them passing through the room. Peace was present, but the feeling of activity all around me was overwhelming. It was something I have never ever felt except the day Heather was hit by the car back in 1989. I knew that feeling, that spiritual being so very present.

I had a flashback to Kyle telling me when Christine came over that she had four babies on her—four babies with different skin colors. He saw babies and children throughout our living room often. He would say, "Mom, the kids are back. They're looking in the windows. They are smiling and waiting for me." I wondered if the children were here in the room at this time. I gave thanks to the Lord, for He is good during this moment—this very moving spiritual moment, the moment that was preparing the way for my son to go to heaven.

People may think I'm crazy, but I could feel the air move by me as they would pass. They would brush my arm. I would tingle with goose bumps and know that God was so very near. Gina felt the presence and saw the white light. There was no car, there was no neighbor to turn on a light, there was no "human" explanation; we knew it was heaven coming down to earth. We knew today was going to be the day. We just didn't know when.

The room was still. Kyle was breathing "normal." Gina was so tired, and I told her to go to sleep. But then I fell asleep on my watch. The Bible story of the disciples falling asleep when Jesus asked them to stay awake came to mind. How could I do that? How did I fall asleep? Was Kyle still breathing?

Not exactly sure why, but I jerked awake. His irregular breathing was what must have startled me awake. He was gurgling in his throat again, that gurgle of death, also known as the death rattle. I got up, called Gina's name, and we both sat with him. The breathing was so bad; this had to be the moment. As our commotion stirred, his breathing became regular again. No, this wasn't going to be the moment he left this earth.

It was about 6:30 a.m., and I needed to get Christian up for school soon. I phoned my sister, and she was going to come and take Christian to school since neither Gina nor I wanted to leave the house for fear Kyle would pass from this life to the next if we left the house.

Christian was getting ready for school, but he didn't want to go. He wanted to stay home. He begged to stay home. He knew something was not right that morning. I lifted him and held him up to his brother's bed. As Christian looked at his big brother, he began talking with him. He told Kyle how much he loved him and that he would see him again one day. I explained to Christian that Kyle was going to be with the Lord very soon in heaven. Christian had known the finality of death. He had witnessed it with my mom just five months earlier. He wasn't going to go to school. He was very strong-willed about staying home. He wouldn't leave his brother. Christian continued to fight me on going to school when Aunt Debbie arrived to take him. He finally kissed Kyle one more time. Tears rolled down my face as I watched my son go off to school. I believed this would be the last time Christian saw his brother alive. Kyle had told me he was going to die while Christian was at school.

CHAPTER 30

Debbie called me after dropping Christian off. Christian had held her hand and said something like "My mom is going to need me today. I want to be with my mom."

Tears streamed down my face. I knew then that Christian knew Kyle was going to die today. Did I do wrong sending him to school? Should he be home? I honestly didn't know what to do. I honestly wasn't sure I made the right decision for him to be at school. How would I handle Kyle's death, let alone help Christian through this time?

The day was passing slowly. Dory called and said she had a turkey dinner for us and would be by about 4:00 p.m. The hospice nurse came, and they had sent an aide to be with us for the day. Family came in and out of the house, with many sitting in the car port. The day was beautiful with the sun shining brightly, and the breeze was blowing gently through the carport, making for a comfortable late summer's day.

Kyle had told me the loved ones he wanted with him when he passed. His respirations were becoming shallow. He had not moved since the strong medications had been administered the day before following his seizure. I made sure and contacted the family he requested. Everyone was present.

Pam, our visiting nurse who had come to our house every week or so to draw blood, arrived at three o'clock. She had received special dispensation to be on his hospice team and visit us once a week to do vitals, etc. This was her day, and she was one of the special people Kyle had requested be with him when he passed.

The nurses exchanged information. Kyle's vitals were slipping. The time was drawing near. I gathered everyone around, and we prayed for him, we kissed him; we spoke private messages of love and "See you soon."

I sat with my boy. An overwhelming feeling of love was over-riding all that was happening, that moment of love, that moment that I knew death was near. I gently touched his beautiful face; it was so thin, and wisps of hair were scattered around his head. My eyes stopped on the top of his head where his pulse was beating out of his skull. My thoughts went back to Kyle as a newborn baby. We were always so careful of his soft spot, and now we were careful once again. That pulse was so strong; the cancer had filled his brain. The beating had been so severe for a couple of days I just silently asked Jesus to take him home. It was time. His very thin arms and legs, chest, and lifeless body were ready to be at rest.

I announced, "Kyle is asking for 'Mom and me time,' just one more time. Just Mom and me. I can feel him desiring time with just me. I'm asking everyone to please step outside." I looked at Fred and asked, "Is that okay?" Tears were welling up in my eyes. I knew Kyle wanted things as they were in the hospital all those months, just "Mom and me," as he always said.

Everyone started to file out of the house and go wait in the car-port. Pam looked at me and said she was *not* going to leave me alone.

"I will be fine. My son wants just me." I assured her I was going to be okay. But I needed this last request granted. Very cautiously, she left and closed the back door.

I sat with my son. I caressed his face. I kissed him.

"Kyle it's just you and Mom. We have our 'Mom and me time.' I am the only one in the house with you. Son, it's time to go be with Jesus. I love you. I will miss you, but I *will* be with you again in heaven!" Tears streaming down my face, I laughed and said, "Son, I tried to promise I wouldn't cry, but know that these tears are tears of joy. I'm so proud of you, the man you have become. The man you have showed others especially during this long cancer journey. The faith you have shown, and the love and placing others above you, especially these last six to eight weeks. It's time, Sweet Kyle with a

Smile. I will love you for always. Go, baby, God is with you. Take the hand of Jesus…"

His body rested; his breathing deteriorated quickly. I called others back inside. Within five minutes, my son took his last earthly breath. He died at 3:35 p.m., exactly when school would end for Christian. As I looked at the clock, I remembered Kyle saying, "I'm going to die while Christian is at school. He's going to need you, Mom." A peace I cannot explain came over me with his last breath.

Pam looked at me and said shortly before this moment something like, "His blood pressure is lowering, be prepared for his heart to keep beating after no more breaths are heard."

Kyle got his request. His eyes were closed. His mouth was closed. His heart stopped beating the moment his last breath was taken. He was in the presence of the mighty Father himself. My son was sitting at the feet of our heavenly Creator or being held in a warm embrace, smiling and being overwhelmed in his beautiful heaven—"Where the grass is a green I've never seen," as Kyle had spoken.

Happy Heaven Day, Kyle Robert. September 19, 2007, 3:35 p.m.

CHAPTER 31

Anneliese wanted to serve her brother one last time. She made sure he was all clean and fresh when Christian came home from school. Kyle was right he would die while Christian was at school. School ended at 3:35 p.m. Darren walked to the bus stop to pick up Christian. He carried him home. Christian had his arms wrapped tightly around Darren's neck; Debbie was with them too. We were all outside, and as Christian looked at me, I knew he knew his brother was in heaven. I mouthed to Darren, "Who told him?" Darren shook his head gently and mouthed, "No one."

I took my little son into my arms and hugged him tightly. Trying not to cry, I sat on the ground under one of our trees, and Christian looked into my eyes eventually and said, "Kyle's with Jesus, isn't he, Mom?" Tears welled in my eyes, and I hugged and hugged him and said, "Yes, he is." We sat for a while, and I just rocked him back and forth.

Then I asked if he wanted to see his brother. We walked into the house, and Kyle lay there so peacefully looking. Christian touched his face, crying and longing to have his brother hug him. We talked about Jesus and how He was holding Kyle for us now. "One day, we will join Kyle again," I promised.

A dear friend brought us a turkey dinner soon after Kyle's passing. She had no clue he would be "gone" upon her arrival. Soon the funeral-home directors arrived, and Kyle was taken from our home. I had to laugh inside and even said, "I'm sorry, buddy. You didn't want to be wrapped up like a Tootsie Roll to go outside the other day, but today you are." He would have loved the humor.

The house was so quiet; the light fall breeze was swishing the trees ever so gently. It was a perfect day, a day Kyle would have loved, a day God brought peace to my son. I thought of Kyle, and I thought of God, with Jesus welcoming him home. "Well done, my good and faithful servant" are words I am sure my son had heard upon his arrival in heaven. Kyle was God's child first, and He loved him more than I could ever imagine! I was so blessed to be chosen as his mom.

CHAPTER 32

Our local paper had followed our story. That evening, the photo editor came to our home to present the audio slide show they had complied with photos Ryan had taken and words they had recorded. He said, "Grab a Kleenex, and let's watch."

My children and I sat ready to watch the video. Christian had been put to bed, and we were all in the living room. I wasn't sure Christian should watch it with us for the first time. I had tucked him in bed and prayed with him. We ended the prayer with "Jesus, please give Kyle a great big hug for us."

One of the balloons that still remained all these weeks from Kyle's "Welcome home" balloons was a GOD LOVES YOU balloon. It kept floating down onto Christian's bed (he slept on the bottom bunk). I would take it by the stem and put it back up on the top bunk. This pattern repeated itself three times.

Christian asked, "Why do you keep moving it?"

"I don't want it to scare you in the night if you happen to wake up."

I went out with the family and began watching the audio slide show. The GOD LOVES YOU balloon came out of the bedroom and into the living room. It hovered just behind the computer, about three feet off the ground. No one said a word; we just watched the slide show and then the balloon. The balloon floated around the living room. It went by each person there. Eventually it went into the kitchen near the stove, where the turkey pan was still sitting, waiting to be washed. The balloon went by Ryan, who was sitting quietly in a corner, watching and observing our reactions to the video and, by now, the balloon too.

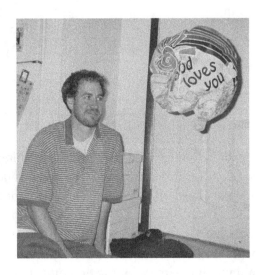

We had fans in the living room blowing, and the balloon defied them. Anneliese said she was turning on the TV to watch *General Hospital* since we had missed the program; the balloon affixed itself to the TV, going right by the air-conditioner fan, blowing the opposite direction.

Gina was in the rocking chair, and it went and bonked her in the head. She started laughing and said, "Okay, okay, Munchy"—her nickname for Kyle—"you can stop hovering!" Kyle would always say that to her as she cuddled and hugged him. They always joked and teased about her "hovering."

That balloon went to each person, and I said, "Okay, Kyle, it's time for bed." It went into my bedroom, and then the boys and came back out to me. I took that balloon in my hands and said, "Thank you, Lord, for showing me my son is with you! It's time for bed now." I carried that balloon into the boys' room and placed it on the top bunk, Kyle's bed, and said, "Thank you, Lord, I love you. And I love Kyle." The balloon never moved again.

Ryan, the photographer, said if he had not witnessed what happened, he never would have believed it. I'm not sure any of us would have, but God had made His presence known that night to each one of us. The balloon chosen out of half a dozen was GOD LOVES YOU. Kyle wasn't present, but God made his personality known to each one of us through that balloon. I slept ten solid hours that night, and the joy of the Lord was so strong!

The audio slide show was released the next day, along with Kyle's passing on the front page of the paper. Many, many, many thousands of people have viewed his testimony around the world. Kyle died way too young by our worldly standards but at the perfect age for God's timing. Our hope is eternal! We must all remember our children are God's first, ours only because he chose us to raise them for Him.

ACKNOWLEDGEMENTS

I wish to thank so many people who have been a part of this journey. I found comfort in the Lord, and from those he sent on our path. Your prayers, helping hands, friendships laughter and tears with my family made a difficult road a little easier to travel down.

My mom, Wanda, was a part of the journey, while she faced her own health issues; she was still a stronghold for me. I believe God took her home five months before Kyle so she could welcome him home to heaven.

My children, you were helpful, loving, encouraging and there as often as you could be during this journey. I am very grateful for all of you. Thank you, Heather & (Brad), Gina Brienne, Anneliese, Darren, and Christian. You are all the biggest blessings in my life. I love you beyond words. I know Kyle cherished each one of you as much as you did him. I couldn't have walked this journey without you all by my side.

My sister Debbie, and her husband, Don were available and there lending a helping hand; through the tears and the laughter. Not only are you my sister, but a friend and shoulder to lean on. Erik, my nephew, but like my seventh child, thank you for lending a hand in so many areas, it was so greatly appreciated. My brother Bob, and wife Sue, along with children Robby and Erin, my brother James and daughter Samantha, thank you for the love and prayers showered on us during our journey. Family is so important, and we all came together. I love you very much.

Thank you also to my cousin, Jennifer, for helping on so many levels, you made life a little easier for us. Peter, Dorie, and family words can't express our gratitude for your wonderful friendship. Peter, you are a special young man, thank you for continuing to include, and visit your friend, as he battled his cancer.

My hospital family: Paul, you were my rock throughout the whole journey! It was a God-incident that we walked our children's journeys at the same time. I am forever grateful for your love and support! Your bear hugs were the best! There are so many other wonderful families we became close to during Kyle's 19 month battle. I won't name each of you, because I will feel bad if I leave anyone out. I love and respect each one of you. From the ones who walked their child to heaven, to the ones still walking on earth, God had a plan and a purpose for all of you!

The hospital staff, again, too many to name, but thank you, thank you, for your service, and love while Kyle was under your care. Marnie, Liz, Carole, Leigh, Kasey are just a few of the super caring nurses that touched Kyle's life in ways that made him feel so special and loved. Jones Soda, yucky jelly beans, slumber parties, monkey bread, and a special visit to him at home, are just a few of the grand memories! The specialists, from oncology, surgical, radiation, etc., were a star team we were blessed to work with! You were all so caring and giving. To each one of you, thank you for treating Kyle so very special, thank you! Dr. Jasty, Dr. Kitchen and Dr. Geiger are three very special physicians that were instrumental in Kyle's care. They will always hold a very special place in my heart.

My community: Neighbors, churches, schools, family, friends, the local newspaper, and strangers thank you for your support on so many levels! Ryan, your photographs are a beautiful portrayal of Kyle's journey that we will cherish forever! Thank you so very much! I love that you captured our hospital days, but also our "normal" days too.

I owe a huge thank you to my cousin, and friend, Christine, and her husband Jeff. They took us on as a mission field, and were there on a moment's notice to care for Christian, drive to the hospital, and so much more. Christine you have encouraged me every step of the way on this journey. You would nudge me to write, to find a publisher, to get Kyle's story out for others to read. You were always there for me, and still are today! Thank you!

Janet, where to begin? You have been my teacher, friend, an encourager, and my biggest advocate for Kyle's journey to become a written testimony for others to hear about. Thank you so much for all of your corrections, suggestions, and especially for believing in me, and that I would bring this project to completion. I will be eternally grateful for the crossing of our paths, and our ongoing friendship! Last but not least, I wish to thank Kyle's dad and step mom. Kyle was one blessed young man to have all of us love him so. I purposefully changed their names for their privacy.

I want to thank God for choosing me to be Kyle's mom. Kyle was/is God's child first, something I needed to remember during our journey. Jesus loved him more than I ever could. I believe Kyle received the ultimate healing, it was God's plan.

Kyle Robert, thank you for being a beautiful soul who left lasting footprints on our hearts; and a contagious smile for everyone who crossed your path. One day we will have "mom and me" time again. I love you!

ABOUT THE AUTHOR

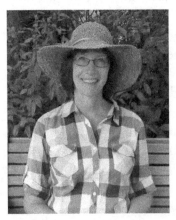

Rebecca Lynn grew up in MidMichigan, where her parents and grandparents demonstrated that God and Jesus were the center of life. She taught her six children, through example, that they can worship God/Jesus at anytime and anywhere because they are ever present.

Her children have given her many "life and death scares" with Kyle's cancer journey being one of the most life-changing she's experienced. She is a strong, compassionate woman, who draws her strength from the Lord. Even through all the struggles she has encountered, she is always ready to lend a helping hand.

Rebecca has had a passion for writing her whole life. She began a school newspaper while in the fifth grade and was editor of her high school news-magazine as a senior. Her dream of being a journalist was pushed aside once she became a mom, but this is when her true gift from God was revealed—to nurture and care for others. Rebecca found comfort in journaling during her life experiences, which led to the writing of *Hope Eternal*.

She has lived in a few different states but can be found today walking the beaches of Lake Huron. She enjoys spending time with her family, which now includes her precious grandchildren.

CPSIA information can be obtained
at www.ICGtesting.com
Printed in the USA
LVHW090230171120
671913LV00018B/91

9 781644 685594